From Cancer to Wellness

the forgotten secrets

a step-by-step handbook for beating cancer

Kristine S. Matheson

Cancer Survivor, Natural Nutritionist, Author, Public Speaker,
Seminar Facilitator, Reiki Practitioner, Angel Intuitive, Artist

Balboa Press books may be ordered through booksellers or by contacting:

Balboa Press
A Division of Hay House
1663 Liberty Drive
Bloomington, IN 47403
www.balboapress.com
1-(877) 407-4847

ISBN: 978-1-4525-4378-9 (sc)
ISBN: 978-1-4525-4379-6 (e)
Library of Congress Control Number: 2011962525

National Library of Australia Cataloguing-in-Publication

Author:	Matheson, Kristine S
Title:	From Cancer to Wellness — the forgotten secrets.
Edition:	1st Edition
Publisher:	Balboa Press
Designer:	Kristine S Matheson
ISBN:	978-1-4525-4378-9 (sc)
Subject:	Beating Cancer
	Cause and Effect
	Alternative Therapy
	Self-Help Step-by-Step Guide

Forgotten Secrets Foundation

www.cancertowellness.com

Important Legal Notice

Dedication

I dedicate this book to my parents, Jean and
Joe Trimbole, for their constant love and support,
and for the faith they have in me to beat
any adversity that comes my way. I am grateful
for the inspiration they have given me to become a
better person and to be true to myself.

Thank you
for everything you have given me
so unconditionally.

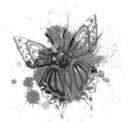

"The journey of life takes us on many twists and turns and along the pathway we look for guideposts to follow. Books can often fulfill this purpose and from the first written words of ancient times to today they have become a storehouse for all the knowledge we need to survive.

Here is a book that we can open to illuminate that pathway to better health and survival in what has become a somewhat hostile environment. Planet earth is polluted, stress is increasing, social conditions are deteriorating, and the economy and climate are more volatile with a host of other factors that are ever present reminders of the fragile nature of human existence.

The ultimate responsibility for good health is not found in our modern health care system but rather, it is each individuals responsibility to equip themselves with information to overcome the greatest epidemic — that of degenerative disease.

This book is a highly valuable asset in presenting clear and concise data that has been successfully applied to guide us to better health, to freedom from degenerative diseases like cancer and to a longer more fulfilling life".

Graham Taylor **ND,BHSc**
Senior Medical Advisor
Living Valley Springs
Kin Kin, Queensland, Australia.

"Kristine Matheson is one of the most positive and courageous women that I have ever known. Having been diagnosed with stage four terminal cancer in 2005, she refused conventional therapy. She gathered all the information available on natural health and nutrition, and then designed her own path to wellness. Her victory has become an inspiration to thousands of cancer sufferers around the world through her enthusiastic public seminars and her motivating book.

Many people, when faced with a crisis, similar to Kristine's 2005 death sentence, give up, break down or retreat into themselves. Kristine did none of these. She courageously challenged herself to learn more about health, and then share her knowledge with the world. She has helped many discouraged victims move forward and take control of their own health, then triumph without the use of drugs or radiation. From that time to the present, she has diligently treated her body as a precious gift from God. She has looked after it with proper nutrition, exercise, sunlight, water, rest and balance.

'From Cancer to Wellness: the forgotten secrets' contains a wealth of information. It is a comprehensive, yet simple guide to anyone who is willing to take the responsibility for their own health.

Kristine is an inspiring and exceptional women. She is a vital advocate in raising awareness of the necessary role of nutrition and natural therapy in the treatment of cancer. Her passion for health education has produced many posisitve results in the national and international communities. She is a giant, a champion, yet humble, unselfish, philanthropic lifesaver who has not only saved her own life, but also the lives of many others."

Gary Martin ND

Founder of Living Valley Springs Health Retreat

Contents

CHAPTER FIVE

CHAPTER SIX

CHAPTER SEVEN

CHAPTER EIGHT

Congratulations!

You have been led to this self-help handbook for a real and exciting purpose:
to change your life and the outcome of your diagnosis.
The bad news is—*Cancer is a reality of life.*
The good news is—*Cancer can be beaten!*

I have done extensive research, which I followed and has contributed to my wellbeing. When you put the information in this book into practice, you will be on your way to a healthier, happier, and more rewarding life, leaving the fear of cancer behind you.

Most of us are searching for better health, happiness and longevity, but it often takes a 'wake up call' to set us on the right track to achieve these goals. This book is an answer to such a wake up call. It is a call to change your direction in life, to avoid an early death, and start enjoying vibrant health and well being. I know you will be able to implement these simple principles daily as you move forward into a better quality of life. Along the way you will meet some amazing people who have overcome the same prognosis as yourself simply by following the guidelines in this handbook.

Most people think the human body has to feel ill to get cancer. This is not true. Healthy and fit people develop malignant cancers without any warning at all. Many of them end up thankful for the journey, which led them into unknown territory that turned out to be valuable to their personal growth and development; I am one of these people myself.

I am not a medical doctor, nor am I a qualified naturopath, yet! I am someone, just like you, who has experienced the fear and reality of being told to *'get your affairs in order'* and *'inform your relatives'* and *'wind down and get ready to die'.*

But, I refused to lie down and die just because an oncologist said I should. After 26 years of study into the prevention and cure of disease, including cancer, I am now studying nutritional and environmental medicine to get my Bachelor degree. I want to put my accumulated knowledge into the hands of those who need it. But I feel so many people need this knowledge now, that I have gone ahead and produced this book prior to my accreditation.

Many people including myself have successfully put into practice the information that is incorporated in this handbook. It is as a result of my success and the success of others that I have been prompted to share this important information. I want to help even more people to come to understand cancer and its effect on people, and for them to know what to do about it.

By putting the information from this book into practice, you can take control of your life, and improve your health.

There are other excellent books on cancer, its causes and cures. I know the program I have developed during years of study and practice will become an easy one for you to follow. Through it you will achieve good health and a valuable lifestyle.

In addition I have experienced chronic fatigue syndrome (CFS), anxiety attacks, business stress, the loss of financial stability and sadly the loss of a child. I am happy to share with you what I have learnt and how I took power over these conditions and situations, and what's more, how I beat terminal stage IV melanoma cancer in a few months. I had been given only twelve months to live, if I was lucky, by an oncologist.

I was 'lucky', for I had a better idea. Instead of submitting my already ailing body to surgery, chemotherapy and radiation, I turned to what I knew, and added to my knowledge so as to find a cure for my condition without medical intervention.

I now pass on this accumulated knowledge to you with love and compassion. I understand the journey you are taking, and I can assure you that there is an answer that can compliment the diagnoses of the medical profession.

I do touch briefly on the way medical practices are not what we are led to believe. However I do not dwell on this negative aspect, or how 'the powers that be' have outlawed cancer cures and promoted drug company interests. There are many books and websites that describe the 'cancer conspiracy' that you may find most interesting and informative. My focus is on you! Getting you well and sharing with everyone how to overcome the disease of the new millennium.

Please give yourself time to read this handbook to the end before making your personal plan for self-renewal, together with a new plan for the remainder of your life. You need a plan that will not only save your life, but also help you enjoy every day in your new lifestyle.

I wish you good health in your personal journey. Please get in touch with me if you need further information. My email is: krissy@theforgottensecrets.com. Embrace the journey you are about to take and most importantly: **Believe in yourself!**

In Health there is freedom!

CAUSE AND EFFECT

The causes of disease are many and varied. The most obvious, from my point of view and after years of research, are:

- lack of good nutrition

- stress

- lack of exercise

- pollution and

- destructive thoughts

Interestingly, according to the medical industry's own findings, the cause of 95 percent of disease is still a mystery. This raises the question: How can the medical profession treat a disease if they do not know the cause?

Millions of dollars are spent on cancer research yearly, without finding a reliable cure. With cell research, microbiological information, nanotechnology, genomic testing, and experience from the past, one would have thought a cure for cancer would have been found by now. The lack of results leads one to ask, "Will they ever find a cure?" and, "If not, why not?" I don't believe they will—not unless some other disease arises to replace cancer and enable research funds to continue to flow into the pharmaceutical industry. They do not see a cure as viable as improving their profitability.

It is not my intention to denounce sincere, practitioners, but the medical profession in general ignores the fundamentals of disease: they ignore the cause. Medical professionals are trained to believe removal of the tumors, followed by chemotherapy, radiation, and drugs is the solution for curing cancer. The * "SPB" (slash, poison, and burn) system is employed immediately after diagnosis by those who assume control of the patient through fear of impending death. The

SPB method does not challenge any of the unanswered questions and hides the mistakes of those in the industry who are intent on using people as guinea pigs.

The answer is simple for those of us who have been through cancer and cured ourselves: return to nature, use natural therapies and alternative thinking, avoid expensive drugs and their many irreversible, painful, and demoralising side effects that kill us in the end.

The drugs used for the SPB method harm the immune system and eventually diminish the body's power to heal itself. SPB kills the good cells with the bad. It also takes power away from the patient and gives it to the professional. Patients treated by SPB are never pronounced "cured." If they do survive the treatments, they are considered in remission. Patients considered in remission are those who have survived and had an extension of life for five years only. On the other hand, those of us who have cured ourselves of cancer know we have overcome the disease and permanently reversed the process. The body has won. Remember, when a tumor is removed by the SPB method, the cancer is not gone. Doctors performing the SPB procedures know this, and so lifelong follow-ups and additional, "just in case" rounds of chemo are required. You become stuck in the "cancer patient" category for the rest of your life. The profession places so much emphasis on the tumor itself, and they know that the cancer cells are still floating around the body. Chasing cancer around your body in order to find it and kill it will eventually kill you. This has been proven over and over again, by the increasing death rate among cancer patients. However, those who have survived to live valuable lives, defying medical treatment and prognosis, tell another story.

It is your choice whether to search and destroy or to bring the body to optimum health so that it can heal itself. This is the fundamental decision you must make: help your body to die or help your body to live. If the human body wasn't a self-healing mechanism, the SPB method might make sense. Giving the body the best chance to heal itself is a better choice, and this choice avoids all the harmful effects brought about by SPB.

The community is conditioned to rely on doctors and scientists for the answers to its ailments. In a perfect world, with honest, humanitarian professionals employing holistic methods of treatment, and trusting the body's capacity to heal itself, their trust would be well founded. Without the drug companies pushing them from behind, this might be possible; unfortunately, this is not so at the moment. We do not live in that perfect world—yet. We live in a world of greed, commercialism, and competition run by those who take advantage of others to keep their research projects going and their drugs coming off the assembly line.

People in the Western world depend too much on doctors and health care professionals. They do not take responsibility for their own body and health care. Surgeons and doctors are trained to "fix" the aftereffects of chronic, degenerative diseases and broken bodies; They receive very limited training in preventive care. Mind you, we no longer live totally in a world of denial and darkness. There are now medical professionals in the world today choosing to educate them themselves further, and implementing nutritional medicine, together with prescribing natural protocols and products for their patients. The number of these doctors is growing. Unfortunately, there are not yet enough doctors practicing this for my liking at this time. When we allow ourselves to be controlled by others instead of maintaining personal responsibility, we become disempowered and take on the fear-based belief systems of those who control us. Maybe this is laziness on our part, or conditioning, or ignorance and a willingness to hand over our power to others. It's easier to take a pill than to change our diet and lifestyle. Or is it? That depends on the outcome you want.

Ty Bollinger writes in his excellent book *Cancer—Step Outside the Box*, "You probably think the true cure rate of orthodox medicine is 40% to 50% and growing rapidly. Nope, it has been 3% for the last 80 years and it isn't going anywhere." I recommend this book, as it contains interesting statistics and valuable information. His message supports the health-promoting program I describe here and will motivate you to make changes in your life.

* SPB Splash Poison Burn — Ty Bollinger, Cancer — Step Outside the Box

Doctors who promote natural healing through diet and nutritional supplements are aware that illness is primarily caused by poor nutrition, stress, lack of exercise, toxicity (pollution), and the way we think. I congratulate medical professionals who are courageous enough to stand up for what they believe about the body's power to heal itself and the importance of proper nutrition, and who do dare fight the system.

Years ago, a general practitioner would never consider recommending physiotherapy, acupuncture, chiropractic, osteopathy, or herbal medicine, and certainly not nutritional supplements and dietary changes. Doctors did not relate nutrition to health. Why not? Because doctors were not taught at university the importance of nutrition or how it relates to disease.

Today, the doctors who are promoting natural nutrition see their patients improving through the value of healing themselves without medical intervention. If you Google "holistic doctors and dentists" or "nutritional and integrative medical practitioners," you will find doctors who choose to heal and prevent disease using methods other than drugs. There are pharmacists who compound bio-identical hormones. They may be able to recommend practitioners who believe in the practice of disease prevention and natural therapies. (A compound pharmacist preparing bio-identical hormones, mixes, and assembles hormone medications from scratch using raw materials, powders customized to suit a particular individual. These hormones are prescribed by a practicing medical doctor).

One doctor describes in his seminars how he left mainstream medicine because he could not continue poisoning his patients with drugs. He was failing to cure them of their illnesses and failing to cure terminal diseases. He says:

> "If you go to the doctor with a headache and the doctor provides you with a prescription for aspirin and the headache goes away, does this mean you have an aspirin mineral deficiency?" (Joel Robbins, *Health Through Nutrition* video, Better Life Products Australia)

We are organic mammals. What goes into our bodies must make up the organic material of which we are made. Yet, nutrition is not taught to most of the medical profession and, therefore, not considered to have any bearing on disease. Only 6 percent of doctors in the United States study nutrition at medical school, and then only as an elective. They are only taught about drugs. Ray D Strand, M.D. *What Your Doctor Doesn't Know About Nutritional Medicine Maybe Killing You* Published 2002.

The first step in combating cancer, or any other environmental disease, is to examine what the body is being fed each day and what it has been exposed to in the past.

The following quote is from the front cover of Herbert Benson's *The Mind/Body Effect* Published 1979: "Don't be afraid to be healthy! As a physician, I am alarmed at the way Americans today are trained to be sick by misguided medical practices. You can improve your health dramatically by learning to trust and rely on your body's own amazing healing powers.". He was associate professor of medicine at Harvard Medical School and director of the Division of Behavioral Medicine at Boston's Beth Israel Hospital.

THE EFFECT OF SUGAR

A REFINED CARBOHYDRATE

One of the first things to remove from your diet PERMANENTELY is sugar.

Sugar is:

Ageing

Fattening

Addictive

A Killer

Sugar raises insulin levels, is a high Glycemic Index (GI) carbohydrate, and causes diabetes, obesity, and most degenerative diseases. Sugar creates fermentation in the stomach and upsets the alkaline balance of the body and the bacteria levels in the gut. Sugar plays havoc with the immune system, leaches out B vitamins, and causes irritability and anxiety.

Many people are seriously ill because they are addicted to sugar. Food manufacturers understand the addictive nature of sugar and promote the consumption of sugar-laden products.

People commonly joke that the cardboard container has more nutrients than most breakfast cereals; but consumers keep eating the cereal because they think if it is allowed to be sold and sitting on the self of the supermarket, then it is safe for them to eat and good for them.

I recommend that you read labels, and I mean ALL LABELS. Ask about the nutritional content of food when buying bulk products, even from health food stores. Many organic processed foods also contain sugar. Remember that sugar is harmful. Be mindful of what you are eating at all times.

Sugar is Cancer Food:

If you have cancer

YOU MUST STOP CONSUMING SUGAR IMMEDIATELY

READ LABELS: READ LABELS: READ LABELS.

Sugar of any kind will feed cancer cells and lead to further growth. Sugar will also add to the excessive growth of candida in the stomach, in those who are susceptible. If you want to survive, sugar has to go. When added to grains and fats, sugar becomes indigestible and blocks the digestive system.

Sugar can be replaced by other herbal substitutes. There are two herbs that I am familiar with that are not harmful to the body. One is Stevia Leaf and the other is Xylitol.

Stevia

Stevia is a member of the chrysanthemum family and comes from the foothills of the Amambay mountain range in Eastern Paraguay, and from Parana State in Brazil. Stevia also grows throughout parts of North America and Latin America. China grows 80% of the world's Stevia leaf, and it has been used for hundreds of years as a sweetener in South America. Stevia is now commercially available all over the world. The Japanese put it in many products, from soft drinks to soy sauce.

It is best to buy stevia in the form of leaves, rather than granules as it is less concentrated. Once stevia is solubilised and crystallised it becomes extremely sweet, 150 to 300 times sweeter than sugar, and with none of the detrimental effects. Stevia is safe for diabetics, is non toxic, and may be used in place of sugar and artificial sweeteners.

People with health problems such as diabetes, obesity, hypoglycemia, high blood pressure, cancer, tooth decay and gum disease, arthritis, candida and digestive problems, to name but a few, will benefit from using stevia. Native Paraguayans and Brazilians enjoy a stevia tea concoction prepared from the leaves, stems and flowers. They boil the leaves in water and then add the thick syrup solution to a variety of drinks to aid digestion, stimulate mental alertness, and regulate blood pressure. This tea also has therapeutic effects on the liver, pancreas and spleen.

Though non-toxic, stevia plants have been found to repel insects, making them ideal for organic gardens. Today, stevia concentrates are marketed in skin care preparations to improve skin tone and remove blemishes. Stevia is also found in dental products, including toothpaste, and mouthwash, and also in pill coatings, pharmaceutical syrups and cough medications. (Extracts from Stevia Facts: www.puresweet.com.au)

Xylitol

Xylitol is a natural sweetener, occurring in many fruits, vegetables and hardwoods. It tastes just like sugar. Xylitol is extracted from birch trees and corn cobs. It has a very low Glycemic Index (GI). Xylitol promotes healthy gums, suppresses helicobacter pylori, and promotes healthy teeth by retarding the demineralisation of tooth enamel. It supports intestinal flora, facilitates intestinal absorption of calcium, helps to maintain bone density, and stabilises blood sugar and insulin levels. All in all, xylitol is a great sugar substitute for those with a 'sweet tooth', and for those who love to bake. Xylitol, looks and feels like sugar, tastes like sugar without the nasty side effects and is alkaline forming in the body. For more information on xylitol, go to www.sweetlife.com.au.

How to stop sugar cravings

If your diet is high in fibre, and includes 80% raw fruit and vegetables as well as fresh fruit juices; this will balance your insulin levels and lower the level of fats in your blood. Adding nut butters, organic eggs, sugar- free yoghurt, brie/ camembert cheeses, and vegetarian proteins to your diet should also reduce blood sugar surges. This will help control cravings, as will barley greens, chlorella, spirulina or kelp, and chromium.

There are other natural substances, like fructose, corn syrup, rice syrup and palm sugar etc. which are promoted as sugar substitutes. However, when they are processed, they break down to sucrose and glucose, or a combination of both, and raise blood triglycerides. Triglycerides are a type of fat circulating in the blood. Raised blood triglycerides are harmful to your health and can lead to heart attacks, strokes and diabetes. You may think it is beneficial to use these sweeteners instead of sugar; but if you have cancer or want to avoid cancer and other diseases, leave them alone.

The only sweeteners to consume are Xylitol, Stevia Later on you may use a little honey; as long as it is raw unpasteurized honey or a little raw organic agave. Agave is great when you are well to add a little to some of the desert recipes. It is still quite a concentrated fructose so needs to be used in very small amounts.

Madjool Dates

Madjool dates are also a good substitute for sweetening desert recipes, smoothies and a great for a small snack. They provide a good source for energy and are full of fibre, vitamins and minerals together with being known to have anti-cancer properties. and to boost immune function.

BEWARE of Poisonous Additives:

Beware also of labels that state "sugar free" as the product may contain Aspartame. This poisonous additive is found in most diet drinks and many diet products. Do not use any artificial sweeteners; they are toxic, cancer-forming and cancer-feeding.

CAFFEINE AND ITS TOXIC EFFECT

Caffeine would be without a doubt the most consumed
and sought after drug in the world today.
Fully active in coffee, tea, chocolate and
many soft drinks being offered to children.

The following extract is from the Australian health retreat, 'Living Valley Springs' (LVS) in 2005 which support my findings and research on the subject of caffeine:

'The US Food and Drug Administration (FDA) have issued a strong warning to pregnant women against the consumption of caffeine because of the possible birth defects. Caffeine has also been related to many areas of disease, such as heart attacks, cancer of the bladder, prostrate, pancreas, ovary, breast cancers and many psychological disorders, not to mention negative effects on the central nervous system, resulting in adrenal exhaustion.

Caffeine also dehydrates the body and a dehydrated body is an acidic body causing blood sugar swings, gastrointestinal problems, nutritional deficiencies and essential mineral depletion.

Calcium Loss

Coffee is linked to loss of calcium in the body. Calcium is an essential mineral that helps the formation of the bones (99% of calcium is located in the bones). When coffee (containing various levels of caffeine from 80–150 milligrams per cup) is consumed, the calcium excreted in the urine increases proportionately with the amount of caffeine that is consumed and in addition, there is an increased excretion of magnesium and sodium in the urine because of the caffeine intake. (Massey and Mondeika, 1984)

Methylxanthines *(rhymes with Ethel Francine)*

Methylxanthines may be vaguely understood by some people and the use of beverages containing this harmful substance such as caffeine, theobromine and theophyllin. This substance causes physical and/or physiological damage. However, it is not well known that these ill effects are serious, sometimes calamitous and may involve any organ or tissue of the body, from scalp to sole. The reason for such widespread damage is found in the chemical nature of Methylxanthines and its ability to alter the very protoplasm of cells, attaching to, or concentrated in cells for an unknown period of time. It should be understood that Methylxanthines are found in coffee, tea, colas and chocolate.

The effects of Methylxanthines begin shortly after taking the drink, food or medication containing them and last about four hours. After eating chocolate or drinking cocoa, you may experience imperfect balance, racing heart, high pitched voice, insomnia, and fatigue and/or finger tremor. Some individuals experience an unexplained sense of dread and anxiety. Other symptoms may be delayed for hours or several days and include sleep disturbances, headaches, restlessness, palpitations, tremulousness, unsteadiness, vertigo, reflex hyper-excitability, irritability, agitation and general discomfort.

Being accustomed to regular intake of Methylxanthines, one may feel less alert, less contented, more sleepy and irritable when there is a delay in drinking the cocoa or eating the chocolate. Many troublesome diseases are made worse by Methylxanthines, e.g. heart disease, allergies, diabetes and fluid retention. They may add to depression and they most certainly contribute to our 'violent society' mind-set. Most gastrointestinal disturbances are aggravated by and some are caused by the intake of Methylxanthines. All Methylxanthines have been associated with chromosome damage and deformities in offspring of the user. Thus: The warning by the FDA for pregnant women to avoid this substance. Cancer is more common in those who have had a regular intake of Methylxanthines resulting in their resistance to disease being seriously reduced.'

Guarana

There is now an influx of 'natural energy' (so called) health drinks, containing a high concentration of caffeine from the plant Guarana. Guarana is produced from the seeds of the Guarana plant, a creeping Amazonian shrub. The black seeds, like an eye, contain a high percentage of caffeine; twice the amount of caffeine than the coffee bean. Used in Brazil as an astringent, a stimulant and often as flavouring, this plant is now being used in many soft drinks and diet products throughout the world and is available in supermarkets and most health food stores and pharmacies. Guarana is also being marketed as a (natural) source of energy.

Reported in the Sydney Morning Herald; the Western Australian Coroner recommended that 'Race 2005 Energy Blast' be removed from the local market after the death of a patient who died suddenly after drinking a quantity of this produce. The product was recalled nationally. This was the second sudden death recorded concerning the intake of this substance.

Just because the label states: 'Natural' or 'Natural Tonic' does not necessarily mean the product is good for you. There needs to be legitimate warnings on all labels, and on all products containing potentially harmful additives. People with underlying health problems need to be able to make informed decisions about what they consume. Anyone with cancer, cardio problems, stress disorders, adrenal fatigue, diabetes, hypoglycemia, and arthritis should keep clear of using products that contain guarana in any form.

Carob

If you love to eat chocolate, the good news is: there is a natural, healthy alternative that is caffeine free and comes from the carob tree. Carob is not an 'empty calorie' food and does not need additives to make it sweet as the carob pods are naturally sweet. Carob is a rich source of pectin, which aids digestion and elimination. Pectin is in the group of indigestible complex carbohydrates commonly called fiber. Pectin in carob is useful for arresting simple diarrhoea, nausea and vomiting and settles the stomach. Like all fibre, pectin helps remove poisons and toxins from the intestines and eliminates them from the body in a natural way.

Lignin is another member of the fibre family found in the 'woody' parts of the carob pod. Both pectin and lignin have a beneficial cholesterol-lowing effect characteristic of dietary fibre.

Beware of any carob product that is sweetened with sugar and made from cow's milk. There are a number of vegan sugar-free delicious products available on the market today; all you have to do is look and ask. Carob also comes in powdered form and makes a great hot beverage for those who enjoy warm drinks.

There are also a number of great recipes you can make if you are looking for a healthy chocolate dessert replacement. If you just cannot live without sweet things, carob is a good choice. Carob chocolate is highly processed; please consume small amounts at a time.

Green tea and White tea

Well known as being part of the cancer fighting regime, 'polyphenols' (often referred to as catechins) in green and white tea are powerful antioxidants that help kill cancer cells. This beverage is 25–100 times more potent than the use of vitamins C and E. Known to also lower bad (LDL) cholesterol and inhibit abnormal formation of blood clots. In recent studies, catechins have shown to fight viruses, slow ageing, destroy free radicals and have far reaching health benefits for the body. Free radicals are highly reactive molecules that can damage the body at a cellular level.

Make sure the quality of the tea you purchase is high grade and is organic; in this way it contains more polyphenols and is more delicious. Unfermented green and/ or white tea leaves are the least processed and this is the most natural way to gain all the health benefits available from these teas.

I recommend you drink three cups of **organic** green tea or white tea every day.

When you're on that coffee date

You need to avoid returning to old habits and thinking *'now I am well, I can have caffeine'*. It is dangerous to think you can go back to your old ways once you are well. In any case why would you want to fall back into fear, heartache, and the risk of ill-health? If you are having a coffee date with friends, and you just cannot resist a coffee, there are many great alternatives that not only taste good, but are good for you.

Organic Dandelion Coffee

Dandelion has long been used as a diuretic. It also helps to lower serum cholesterol and uric levels. Known also to be supportive by improving kidney function. It also is most beneficial in the prevention and treatment of breast cancer. Dandelion is full of phytochemicals and nutrients.

Ganoderma Lucidum Coffee

Ganoderma Lucidum, or Reishi Mushroom as it is commonly referred to, not only tastes like real coffee, it is also alkaline-forming in the body, raising your pH level, rather than bringing it down. When buying Ganoderma coffee make sure the caffeine content is minimal only 8–19 mgs per cup, in comparison to 80–150mg of caffeine in regular coffee, 40–80 mg in ordinary black tea, and 46 mg in Coca Cola. Normal coffee has a pH level of 5.5; Ganoderma Coffee if it is low in caffeine should have a neutral pH reading between 7.3 and 7.5. Always inquire about the active ingredients in all purchases. One company stating the caffeine content in their products is approximately nil (or a maximum of 17mg per cup) is Gano Excel.

Reishi mushroom is a valuable herb, used throughout Asia for over 4000 years for medicinal purposes, and has been commonly used to fight cancer. The Reishi mushroom contains polysaccharides, which strengthens the immune system, and germanium, which increases oxygen in the blood. It also contains 200 active elements known to improve health, including 165 antioxidants.

Apart from its alkalising effect on the body, the Reishi Mushroom is known to improve sleep, help balance weight, increase oxygen to the brain, and boost overall health by removing toxins from the system. The Reishi mushroom has been known to also assist in the cure of arthritis and diabetes.

It is recommended to drink Ganoderma coffee black when fighting cancer.

Ganoderma Lucidum Tea

Organic Ganoderma Lucidum tea tastes similar to ordinary black tea, but does not have the bad side effects. Ganoderma tea is often used to relieve nausea in cancer patients who have been treated with chemotherapy and radiation. The other benefits of this product are the same as for Ganoderma coffee. There is no caffeine or tannin in this tea.

Cacao - raw

Most of us like real chocolate. The problem is those who are addicted to chocolate are acutually addicted to the sugar and caffeine.

We often see segments on television or read in magazines, the benefits of chocolate because of the high antioxidant levels. I often get a little frustrated when hearing or reading this because very few people telling the story give you all the facts.

Firstly it is the raw cacao bean that is healthy not processed cocoa. See how differently it is spelt. It is raw cacao that is high in antioxidants that benefit us in general whole body health. In processed dark chocolate, antioxidants such as epichatehins, chatechins, resveratrol and procyanidins can be present, but are in much lower levels than in unheated raw chocolate. Not only do most raw chocolate bars taste delicious, they are generally sweetened with stevia, xylitol or agave, not sugar. Making deserts with raw cacao nibs and powders are also delicious and good for us. Raw cacao is caffeine free and safe to consume. To find out more about this amazing food go to www.sacrededenblog.com/cacao-and-benefits.

THE EFFECT OF ALCOHOL

$\mathcal{J}$UST ONE DRINK WON'T HURT ME! — OR WILL IT?

If you are trying to avoid cancer or cure yourself of cancer then
ALL ALCOHOL must be avoided.

$\mathcal{R}$esearch shows that drinking alcohol for over twenty years or more can cause cancer of the mouth, throat, esophagus and liver. Also, alcohol affects estrogen levels in men and women who are susceptible to breast cancer. In 2008, the International Agency for Research on Cancer added breast and colon cancer, two of the four major killers, to the list of malignancies known to be fostered by alcohol.

The Mediterranean diet is known to reduce coronary heart disease, prevent diabetes and reduce the chance of premature death. The Mediterranean diet includes the daily consumption of red wine. The relaxation effect of wine alone is beneficial. Many people living with too much stress drink alcohol to relieve the pressures of life. But alcohol is not the answer. It is far better to meditate, go for leisurely walks, do some yoga, listen to relaxation CD's, watch a funny movie, and so forth. The benefits of these activities far outweigh those of wine drinking.

The skin and seeds of grapes used to manufacture good wine are rich in proanthocyanidins, an antioxidant flavonoid that removes free oxygen radicals from cells. Grape seeds contain a high concentration of these antioxidant flavonoids and are now being marketed worldwide as a dietary supplement. The problems with wine are alcohol and the preservatives sulphur dioxide and sodium sulphite (220, 221) especially for those suffering the effects of cancer. The alcohol in wine puts stress on the liver, is a depressant, destroys brain cells, and destroys B vitamins, which in turn, harms the immune system. The preservatives are also toxic to the liver, destroying vitamin A and B, all of which are important for good health and keeping the nervous system functioning correctly.

Alcohol, impairs your thinking, causes headaches, ferments in the stomach, and is extremely dehydrating. It can disturb your sleep and affects meditation and relaxation techniques. Alcohol leaves you with less control over your actions and choices, distorting your perception of reality. This can lead to you making bad food choices, and cravings for something sweet.

Organic wine

Do not be deceived by the word 'organic' on wine labels. The effects of alcohol are the same. Strangely enough, many organic wineries add preservative to their wine. I am amazed that they take the trouble to grow organic grapes and then destroy their product with toxic preservatives. Organic products are supposed to be better for you. Manufacturers use the word 'organic' and consumers presume their product is of high quality and good for you. It is important to read all labels when manufacturers advertise organic or chemical free on their products, no matter what you buy. The wine industry claims the preservatives give the wine a longer shelf life. Alcohol itself is a preservative, so why does it need additives?

De-alcholised wines

De-alcholised wines have most of the alcohol removed leaving only about one half of one percent. This does not mean it is better for you. The preservative sulphur dioxide is added to all the brands I have found. The fermentation process is the same and the wine is acid forming in the stomach.

I would love an occasional glass of wine

I suggest that if you enjoy a glass of wine, you should do so occasionally, and only when you are cancer free. Buy either bio-dynamic or kosher wine. These two types I have been told do not use chemicals in the processing or the bottling. It is important to enquire if preservative has been added before choosing a wine. If you do have the occasional glass of wine, make sure you do not exceed one glass, and drink plenty of water.

Even one glass is dehydrating and acid forming.

FATS AND OILS

Ⓗow do they effect the body?

'OILS JUST AIN'T OILS—FATS JUST AIN'T FATS EITHER'

You need to know the difference!

There are good fats—fats that heal.

There are bad fats—fats that can send you to an early grave.

Ⓣhe bad fats that are found in the modern western diet have been linked to cancer, especially skin, breast, pancreatic and colon cancer. Like sugar and refined carbohydrates, bad fats, cause degenerative disease, such as heart disease, diabetes, hypoglycemia, arthritis and lifestyle conditions such as obesity. Bad fats are indigestible, creating excess cholesterol which is stored in the blood and tissues.

Good fats and oils from cold pressed extraction which are grown organically, are essential to our daily diet for the health of our central nervous system (our brain being 60 per cent fat). Fats protect our vital organs. Fats and oils deserve a book on their own. An excellent book to read is 'Fats That Heal, Fats That Kill' by Udo Erasmus — published by Alive Books, Canada.

The French

'The French are healthier, fitter and live longer than populations of most countries. Is it genetic? It is interesting to note that studies have shown that Americans who move to France lose weight, get fitter and healthier and live longer. So what is it that gives France the edge?

Fast food stores and supermarkets are not common in France. Food is fresh and often locally grown. Even the smallest brasserie would never cook with dehydrated or frozen foods. The French eat small to moderate meals, ensuring maximum nutrition in each preparation. Whereas, the Americans have 3–4 times the volume per meal. The French stop eating when no longer hungry, whereas the Americans and Australians tend to stop only when their plate is clean. The French consume more fat than any other nation on Earth, ingesting 170gms per person per day, against a world average of 78gms.' (Food & Ag org of UN. www.fao.org/statistics/yearbook/ vol_1_1/site_en.asp?page+C)

A doctor Serge Renaud from the Bordeaux University coined the term "French Paradox" in 1992 when he determined that saturated fats make up the majority of the 170gms.

In his book 'The Fat Fallacy', Dr Will Clower suggests that the paradox may be narrowed down to a few key factors. The French eat good fats as opposed to bad fats. They get up to 80% of their fat from dairy and vegetables sources. They eat butter (4 times more than Americans), soft cultured cheeses such as camembert, brie and blue vein, cream, sour cream and yoghurt. They do not eat margarine, trans fats, hydrogenated fats or refined oils. They eat their food slowly. They do not snack between meals. The French avoid products that contain sugar. They prefer full-fat foods rather than processed low-fat foods'. (ref: Gary Martin ND — Lifestyle Excellence May–July 2009)

The Good Fats

- **Monounsaturated Fats:**

  These fats lower total LDL (bad) cholesterol and increase HDL (good) cholesterol.

  Some foods that contain monounsaturated fats are:

  ✔ **Nuts** — almonds, macadamias, walnuts, hazelnuts, peanuts, pistachios.

  ✔ **Vegetable Oils** — avocado oil, olive oil, peanut oil, sunflower oil, sesame oil.

- **Polyunsaturated Fats:**

  These fats lower total LDL (bad) cholesterol.

  Foods that are high in polyunsaturated fats include:

  ✔ **Nuts and seeds** — walnuts and sunflower seeds.

  ✔ **Vegetable oils** — soybean oil, corn oil, safflower oil, linseed oil, hemp seed oil.

  ✔ **Seafood** — salmon, herring, trout, mackerel and fish oil. Omega 3 fatty acids are included in this group.

The Bad Fats

- **Saturated Fats**

  Saturated fats raise LDL (bad) cholesterol.

  Foods that are high in saturated fat are:

  ✗ **Animal products**—beef, pork, lamb, veal, lard, poultry fat, cream, milk, yellow cheeses and some other dairy products.

  ✗ **Plants**—palm oil, palm kernel and cocoa butter.

  I have not included eggs, butter, white cheeses and coconut oil, although they are saturated fats; I believe them to be safe and healing to the body.

- **Trans Fatty Acids**

  Trans fatty acids raise LDL (bad) cholesterol and are cancer forming.

  Some foods contain trans fats as a result of the hydrogenation of liquid oil. They include:

  ✗ **Commercially packaged foods**—fried foods, all margarines, shortening, fast foods, packaged snacks, crackers, biscuits, cookies, doughnuts, muffins, pies, cakes, and processed meat products.

How to choose

What I wish to impress upon you, is how to use oils and fats and which ones **ONLY** to use.

Many fats and oils are being marketed as 'low fat', 'low cholesterol' on the label or container. These fats are supposedly good for your health, don't believe it, this is misguided information.

Highly processed, hydrogenated, overheated oils and margarines are BAD for you and are extremely rancid. I cannot say how BAD they are! It has been said for example that margarine is only one molecule away from being 'plastic'!

If you must add fat to your bread, soups, or any other foodstuff, use 100% organic butter, ghee, organic cold pressed olive oil, organic nut butters, or avocado.

There are only a few oils stable and safe enough to use in cooking, because of their tendency to become rancid when heated.

Become familiar with the following list of oils as a guide to cooking safely.

HEAT STABLE	MODERATELY STABLE	UNSTABLE
COCONUT	SESAME	SUNFLOWER
BUTTER/GHEE	PEANUT	CORN
MACADAMIA	HAZELNUT	LINSEED
	ALMOND	
	OLIVE	

NB: All Oils must be produced by organic cold pressed extraction.

Organic coconut oil

Although this is a saturated oil which we have been told in the past to avoid, it has since been discovered that coconut oil has many healing benefits. It is good for the heart as it lowers cholesterol. Coconut oil is also excellent for those suffering diabetes, as well as preventing and treating thyroid-related ailments. Coconut oil also helps maintain a healthy scalp and hair; and most importantly, it is anti-carcinogenic. Coconut oil has been shown to reduce and even eliminate tumors; and it does not go rancid when heated to a high temperature. Putting two tablespoons in your warm lemon drink first thing in the morning, together with vitamin C is very palatable.

Coconut oil is now being used in some countries for commercial cooking, because of its benefits to general health. Together with organic cold pressed olive oil, coconut oil needs to be added to your daily intake of nutrients. Go to www.nuicoconut.com and www.thaiorganiclife.com for further information.

Apart from the above benefits for this exceptional oil, it can be used in place of a moisturizer, a hair and scalp conditioner, and for sun protection due to its antioxidant properties. Some oils on the body make your skin burn; it would seem that the oil you place on your body is just as important as the oil you put in it. Virgin coconut oil when being employed with an anti candida program, and a weight loss program is extremely beneficial.

Omega 3 (EPA/DHA)

Omega 3 is polyunsaturated oil with components of Linolenic Acid that convert to EPA/DHA, two long chain fatty acids needed for brain function, and essential to mental and cardiovascular health. Linolenic Acid protects arteries from damage, reduces triglycerides, and lowers LDL cholesterol. It also inhibits blood clotting, lowers blood pressure, and reduces the risk of heart attack and strokes. Omega 3 is also an anti-inflammatory and is used to prevent osteoarthritis, and is used in the treatment of rheumatoid arthritis, and autoimmune disease, and in the prevention and treatment of cancer. Cells need omega 3 acids to oxygenate properly. These oils are mainly found in marine animals such as sardines, cod, tuna, mackerel, eel, anchovy, pilchards, cold water trout, and salmon. A healthier and more humane way to get your Omega 3 is from Algae.

Algae—the healthier alternative

Flaxseed and hemp oils are often recommended sources of omega 3 for those who follow a vegetarian or vegan diet. Omega 3 in this form provides a limited conversion to EPA and does not convert at all to DHA when ingested. Vegan sources of omega 3's that do convert to DHA are found in algae extractions.

Algae are one of the oldest food sources on the planet and used by the ancient Aztecs and Chinese for its prophylactic properties and does not contribute to the world's diminishing fish stocks. By comparison, it takes 500kg of fish bodies to make just 1kg of fish oil and manufacturers are now catching fish simply for the oil content, which is decimating global fish stocks and upsetting the entire food chain (Ref: Water 4 Investments Ltd).

Algae-derived compounds prevent cancer cells from spreading; together with a good diet, will also shrink tumors. An excellent inexpensive organic product called Deva Omega-3 DHA is available worldwide. Go to www.devanutrition.com for online or store availability.

We consume too much omega 6 nowadays which includes fast food; too much processed grains, meat and poultry, and hydrogenated, unsaturated fats that destroy the omega 3 active components. Subsequently, the use of supplementation, particularly omega 3 with the ratio of 3 (omega 3) to 1 of omega 6, seems to be necessary.

Max Gerson, a cancer researcher in the 1950's, developed nutritional protocols and a successful detoxification that cured most cancers. He used omega 3 oils in the treatment of cancer and other degenerative diseases

Today, omega 3 in the diet is being used to prevent disease. It is also given for the treatment of cancer, arthritis, (osteo and rheumatoid), heart disease, angina, bile and pancreatic problems, celiac disease, diabetes, chronic fatigue and is also beneficial in lowering elevated triglycerides and cholesterol, decreasing the LDL's. Omega 3 can also help with inflammatory problems, immune disorders, stress, and blood disorders. It is used to support premature babies, obesity, Parkinson's disease, alcoholism, MS (multiple sclerosis), gall bladder disease, skin disorders (including eczema, psoriasis and acne), and other debilitating diseases can all be treated with omega 3.

PROTEIN

$\mathcal{H}$ow important is protein?

and

What type is best to consume?

Protein is essential along with a variety of fresh fruit,
vegetables and whole foods, to achieve a balance of
vitamins, minerals, trace elements and amino acids
for cell regeneration and healing.

$\mathcal{T}$he best type of protein comes from concentrated organic plants. These include a variety of pulses and legumes — lentils, chick peas (also known as garbanzos), beans, red kidney beans, lima beans, pinto, black beans, white beans, butter beans, borlotti beans, haricot beans, cannellini beans, navy beans, adzuki beans, split peas, nuts and seeds. These should be combined with grains such as rice to make a 'complete protein'. Fermented soy products such as tempeh, miso, and tofu are all complete proteins and contain higher nutrients than standard food products, for example, glutathione, a major antioxidant needed to synthesize all other antioxidants in the body, and B-vitamins. Protein can be found in some vegetables. Some of the vegetables that contain protein are; mushrooms, coconut, corn, peas, spirulina, algae, barley greens and wheat grass.

Legumes and beans are known to inhibit the overgrowth of yeast in the body. They nourish the intestine, cells, reduce cancer development, and they decrease LDL cholesterol, thus reducing the risk of heart disease and diabetes. They also prevent constipation and many bowel diseases. It is best to sprout all legumes, beans and nuts.

Legumes and beans can cause gas if they are not soaked overnight or for at least 4 hours before cooking. This helps break down the starches and aids in digestion. Wash the legumes two or three times, and then cook in fresh filtered water.

Cooking does cause, however, the amino acids in protein to coagulate. The body has to work harder to extract amino acids when protein is cooked. It is better to consume proteins raw by sprouting legumes and beans.

Commercial, non-organic beans and legumes are toxic. There is a chemical residue from harvesting and processing. When choosing canned beans and legumes, select organic brands to non-organic brands; they are inexpensive, and a staple food well worth using when your time is limited.

Soaking nuts for 24 hours before eating makes them more digestible. Almonds should have their skins removed after soaking, as they are slightly toxic. If you forget to soak almonds, blanch them in boiling water for 60 seconds, and the skins will come off easily.

To ensure you get all the essential amino acids you need in one meal, you need to combine vegetarian sources as described below, to form a complete protein.

Combine **Legumes, beans, peas with <u>one</u> of the following: grains, wild or brown rice, nuts, seeds, corn.**

OR

Combine **Wild or brown rice with <u>one</u> of the following: beans, nuts, seeds, grains.**

Although I lean towards being a vegan, I do think it is necessary for those who wish to remain healthy to consume organic eggs, organic butter, organic white cheeses such as brie and camembert, and organic yoghurt; in this way you can be assured of a healthy balanced diet and avoid being deprived of B12.

If you have difficulty absorbing B12 or wish to live a vegan lifestyle, B12 is available in a liquid form and can be taken under the tongue using a dropper. Also available is tablets that are dissolved in the cheek, this is a sublingual form of taking B12. The best sublingual B12 to use for greater absorption is 'Methylcobalamin'. Also available are vitamin B12 and Multi B injections that can be ordered from your medical practitioner and administered in their surgery. Injections are inexpensive and worthwhile. See section on sprouting for a list of living foods that contain vitamin B12.

Yoghurt

Make sure yoghurt is not sweetened or flavoured and does not contain preservatives. Use only organic or bio-dynamic yoghurt; sweeten it yourself with fresh fruit juice, fresh fruit, stevia, or xylitol. Yoghurt is a complete protein, rich in potassium and B vitamins, especially B2, B12, and folic acid. Yoghurt contains all the friendly bacteria needed for digestion.

Yoghurt also prevents and helps to cure candida. It helps to fight infection by improving the immune system. The best yoghurts, in my opinion, are made from sheep or goats milk. Do not consume if you are allergic to or intolerant to dairy.

Eggs

For some time, eggs have had a bad name. Some health experts say they are too high in cholesterol. Gary Martin ND disagrees as this can be seen in this extract from Lifestyle Excellence "Cholesterol", March–April 2006. P1:

'It is not the eggs, butter, sour cream, brie and camembert that harden the arteries. It is the acid forming foods such as sugar, refined grain foods, soft drinks, fast foods etc. that change the pH of the blood. In response to acidosis, the bones secrete phosphates to neutralise acids. Calcium is subsequently released into the blood where it binds to cholesterol (LDL). This combination forms plaque'.

'Preparation for elimination can be enhanced by increasing protein, particularly organic eggs, and taking antioxidants such as Vitamin A, C and E, Glutathione, Co-Enzyme Q10, Selenium, Quercetin, Zinc and Phyto nutrients such as Brassica vegetables, St Mary's Thistle, Green tea and Lemon Peel'—(Gary Martin ND, Detoxification—Web Link—Resources Page 2).

If you are not allergic to eggs, include them in your diet — poached of course or soft boiled; avoid fried and hard boiled eggs; remember ORGANIC, ORGANIC, ORGANIC.

Non organic eggs come from caged battery hens which are made to suffer inhumane conditions. Always choose 'Certified Organic Free Range' eggs. Chickens in cages have their beaks trimmed so they do not attack each other. They do not have freedom to spread their wings, nor live any kind of natural life. They are injected with antibiotics and with hormones and steroids. They are fed the remains of their own kind, and are void of B12 and almost every other nutrient. The flesh of the chicken and the eggs are not at all good for human consumption.

Even so called 'Free Range' eggs from 'free range' chickens are not to be trusted for their quality and nutritional value. The birds are often housed in huge sheds without freedom to move far. The only difference between their conditions and those of battery hens is that there is no cage. They are still standing in cramped, unnatural conditions.

Certified organic eggs on the other hand, are from hens that roam freely and are fed on grains which were organically grown. The hens enjoy their natural diet of insects and grubs and they are not fed chemicals or hormones. They are not injected with antibiotics, nor are they caged or confined in breeding sheds. Before buying organic eggs, check that they have been certified by a registered certifier in your country of origin. This means they will be labeled with a certification logo.

Cheese

Avoid hard, yellow cheeses — these contain saturated fats, colourings, chemicals, processed table salt, and synthetic vitamins. People joke about 'plastic cheese' and yet they still eat it! Small amounts of organic cottage cheese, brie or camembert can usually be tolerated, as long as you do not have an allergy to dairy products

NB: In the following page I will tell you to stay away from dairy. This might confuse you as I have mentioned it is OK for you to have a little yoghurt or white cheese. Yoghurt and white cheeses are fermented in a way that makes it easy for digestion and they are sometimes helpful when and if you go through a healing crisis. These foods sometimes relieve headaches. Do not consume large amounts though and if allergic or intollerant to dairy avoid altogether.

Cow's Milk and Dairy Products

These are mucus forming, and often the cause of allergies, such as asthma, dermatitis, eczema, sinusitis, post nasal drip. Dairy food can cause other problems, such as middle ear infections, arthritis, heart disease, migraine headaches, malabsorption of nutrition, diarrhoea, constipation and hormone imbalances, to name but a few.

The proteins in milk strip the calcium from the body. If you are worried about where you will get your calcium from, a question I am often asked, there are many other sources. You will find some in the recipe section.

The only milk from an animal suitable for human consumption is human milk. Humans are the only mammals that drink another animal's milk. Do not drink cow's milk; it is indigestible and harmful to your recovery. Drink other forms of organic sugar free and malt free milk such as, rice, almond, oat, cashew and above all coconut milk.

Eighty percent of people are intolerant to lactose — an enzyme in cow's milk. Consuming food that cause an allergic or intolerant reaction puts a strain on the immune system. Casein is a protein in dairy and many people are also allergic to this and are unaware they have this problem. Allergies are the immune systems response to an environmental substance, foods, plants or animals.

Bee Pollen

These are rich sources of protein and vitamin B12, multi B vitamins, essential fatty acids, vitamin C, carotene, calcium, iron, magnesium, enzymes, potassium, manganese, sodium, plant sterols, and simple sugars; they are known to be a complete food containing nearly all the nutrients we require.

Bee pollen has been used in Chinese culture for centuries for many forms of healing, and for its ability to enhance endurance and vitality. Bee pollen is used as a cure for cancer as it kills tumor cells, and for its antiviral properties in treating of chronic fatigue syndrome (CFS), depression and some colon disorders.

Bee Pollen is used in the treatment of fungal infections, for healing ulcerated sores, and other skin disorders. Buy only raw unpasteurized organic products.

Protein Powders

From time to time you may need to use protein powders. If you do so, particularly if you are experiencing headaches while your body is detoxing, use only **raw (unde-natured)** protein powders.

Raw (unde-natured) protein powder supports the immune system, with immunoglobulin's and lactoferrin; they also increase glutathione, which is the body's main free radical scavenger. It has the ability to detoxify the cells and support cellular repair and is a very digestible source of protein. Make sure you purchase **only** raw (unde-natured) protein powders. De-natured products have been heated, and have lost certain immune-enhancing ingredients.

Garden of Life Raw Protein Powder

Garden of Life Raw Protein is for anyone who wants to add a premium-quality organic vegan protein and/or super nutrition to their diet. It includes the nutritive power of certified organic living seeds and grains. Featuring 13 raw and organic sprouts, and is an excellent source of protein plus essential amino acids. Raw Protein supports the digestive health and function with live protein-degesting enzymes and powerful probiotics. To find your nearest stockist go to www.gardenoflife.com. This product is also available through www.iherb.com

Garden of Life products are made in the United States, and are my favorite brand for protein powders. The also have a Raw Meal containing 26 superfoods, raw organic spouts, seeds and greens. This is a great addition to your daily program, especially if you are needing to stabilize your weight.

Other Highly Recommended Protein Powders:

Sun Warrior Unde-natured Organic Rice Protein

Sun Warrior Protein is a raw, vegan protein powder produced from fermented raw wholegrain brown rice. The rice has been germinated to maximise bioactivity. It is easy to digest and is 85% pure protein. Sun Warrior also contains high quality amino acids which the body can easily absorb, including lysine, and other essential vitamins and minerals. Available through internet stores and health food stores, Sun Warrior is produced in the United States.

ImmunoPro and RenewPro Unde-natured Whey Protein

These two whey protein powders are high in antioxidants, with high levels of lactoferrin and other anti-cancer immune properties. They support detoxification, and are easily digestible and support the body's fight against cancer.

Raw Power Protein Superfood

Raw Power Protein Superfood Blend is a combination of hemp protein powder, and Brazil nut protein powder that contains 50% protein and provides antioxidant benefits with its high selenium content. This blend also contains maca powder, goji berry powder, mesquite powder, maca extreme which is a potent form of maca in the world. Available through Internet stores and some health food stores and cafes. To buy online go to www.rawpower.com

$\mathcal{P}$rotein needed for regeneration of cells

Do not be misled into thinking that you require huge amounts of protein; this is not the case. This is misinformation put out by the meat industry. Researchers believe, on average, we need approximately 2% to 4% of protein from the intake of calories per day. The amount required by each person will depend on their weight, age, state of health and level of activity. The average person consumes 15% to 20% of protein per day which is a far cry from what researchers believe is necessary. Also researchers have shown that this protein can quite successfully come from vegetarian sources. John Toomey, a conditioning coach and nutritionist working at the elite level in Australian sport says when referring to athletes, and I am sure he would agree that this statement is correct for all humans, '*Athletes need life force. You cannot get life force from a dead animal*'.

Discuss your protein requirements with your health-care provider if you feel the need. Bearing in mind, to eliminate cancer, you will need to maintain a vegetarian diet. See Program for Life and Recommended Optimum Daily Program in this handbook.

A vegetarian diet containing fresh vegetables, legumes and whole grains together with certified organic eggs, cultured dairy products, such as yoghurt and white cheeses the best being Brie and Camembert, together with organic butter has enough protein to heal the body and maintain good health. A diet of red meat, farmed fish, non-organic chicken, and dairy products cause disease and are very acidic. This type of protein does not cure disease!

ARE YOU ACID OR ALKALINE?

and

$\mathcal{W}$hat does this mean?

The food and drink we consume is either alkaline or acid-forming.
The more acid our body, the more susceptible we are to disease and ill health.

An acidic body does not absorb vitamins, minerals and other nutrients and reduces our ability to repair cells. Cancer thrives in an acidic body. On the other hand, an alkaline body heals and repairs cells and absorbs nutrition. Cancer also hates oxygen, and if the body is alkaline the body is more oxygenated therefore, cancer cells cannot survive.

Not only do the foods and liquids we eat and drink determine pH levels, so do stress and pollution.

So what foods should you eat to stay alkaline? Most raw fruits and vegetables metabolise in the body, leaving an alkaline residue. If we eat 80% raw and 20% cooked food, drink plenty of alkaline water, and reduce stress, you will remain alkaline.

It is commonly believed that this percentage can be changed to 60% raw and 40% cooked. However, it is best to keep with the 80–20 ratio to be and remain cancer free. Once you have been restored to health, it is acceptable to adopt the 60–40 regime, **but only on occasions.**

The juice of half a lemon in a glass of water three times a day will also help the body to become alkaline (see Program for Life). Drinking lemon juice first thing in the morning with warm (not hot) water opens all the little capillaries in the digestive system in readiness to absorb nutrition. Limes are as good as lemons.

Super foods, such as green barley, wheat grass, maca, and bee pollen are alkaline-forming in the body and so help reduce acidity. Lactates found in cultured foods such as yoghurt, sauerkraut, Brie and Camembert cheeses, also reduce acidity.

The body must have a pH reading between 7.35–7.45 in order to be alkaline. This is a safe range for healing. Too much acidity kills. Too much alkalinity (over 8.1) may cause health problems; remaining too alkaline for a long period of time can kill too. It is important to your health to keep a balance.

The pH scale below is from 4.5 to 11.0 and shows the healthy range

4.5 5.0 5.5 6.0 6.5 7.0 Healthy Alkaline 8.0 8.5 9.0 9.5 10.0 10.5 11.0

You must test your pH daily particularly if you have cancer.

How do you test your pH?

- Put some saliva or urine on a piece of pH paper, commonly known as Litmus Paper.

- Wait thirty seconds and compare the colour of the paper with the colour of the scale on the pH paper dispenser.

- You need to do this when you wake up before eating or drinking.

- Test again two hours after breakfast.

- You can also test, just before going to bed. Again, this should be done two hours after eating or drinking.

I recommend you buy pH paper from your local pharmacy, drugstore, or health food store. You can also get it from health care practitioners, but at a higher cost.

Micro Essentials have an excellent product you can buy direct. The small plastic dispenser it comes in protects the paper from humidity, and is very easy to use with very little wastage. To buy pH papers direct go to www.microessentiallab.com;

All pharmaceutical drugs, artificial sweeteners, tobacco, caffeine, processed food and beverages are highly acidic. All products need to be organic/chemical free to avoid pesticides which are acid.

The following food and beverages are **ALKALINE-FORMING** in the body.

Vegetables (raw) — alfalfa, artichoke, asparagus, barley greens, beetroot, beet greens, broccoli, brussels sprouts, beans(green), cabbage, carrot, cauliflower, celery, chives, chlorella, corn, cucumber, dulce, dandelion, daikon, eggplant, grasses (wheat, straw, barley, kamut etc.), kale, kombu, lettuce, maitake mushrooms, nori, onions, parsnips, peas, peppers, potatoes (dry baked in their skins), pumpkin (dry baked in their skins), radish, red cabbage, reishi mushrooms, sauerkraut, sea vegetables, shitake mushrooms, spinach, spirulina, sprouts, squash, swedes, turnips, wakame, watercress.

Fruit (raw) — apples, apricots, avocados, bananas, blackberries, blueberries, cantaloupe, cherries, coconut — fresh, currants, dates, figs, grapes, grapefruit, mangos, lemons, limes, nectarines, oranges, papaya, peaches, pears, pineapples, raisins, raspberries, rock melon, strawberries, tangerines, tomatoes, umbroshi plums, watermelon.

Protein — almonds, brazil nuts, chestnuts, chick peas (sprouted), eggs (raw), flax seed, lentils (sprouted), lima beans, millet, pumpkin seeds, rice protein powder (raw), soured dairy products, sesame seeds, sunflower seeds, tofu (fermented), tempeh (fermented), whey protein powder (raw).

Beverages — alkaline mineral water, banchi tea, dandelion tea, fresh fruit juices, ganoderma coffee (black), ganoderma tea, ginseng tea, green juices, green tea, herbal teas, kombucha, vegetable broth, vegetable juices (fresh), white tea

Oils and fats — avocado, borage, coconut oil, evening primrose, flax, hemp, olive, and udo oil.

Others — all herbs, apple cider vinegar, bee pollen, Celtic salt, chili powder, cinnamon, cumin, curry, ginger, honey (raw unpasteurized), horseradish, hummus, lecithin granules, maple syrup, miso, molasses, sea salt, sprouted seeds, stevia, tamari, tahini, xylitol.

The following foods are ACID FORMING in the body:

Fruit & vegetables—cranberries, fruit cooked and canned, olives, plums, potatoes—cooked (except dry baked in their jackets), prunes, vegetables cooked and canned.

Animal protein—bacon, beef, carp, chicken, clams, corned beef, eggs, fish, ham, kidney, lamb, liver, lobster, mussels, oysters, pork, processed meats, rabbit, salmon, sardines, sausages, scallops, shellfish, shrimp, tripe, turkey, veal, venison.

Beverages—all alcoholic drinks, beer, black tea, coffee, cocoa, commercial fruit juices, hard liquor, smoothies, soft drinks, wine.

Oil and fats—canola oil, corn oil, hydrogenated oils, margarine, and vegetable oil saturated fats, sunflower oil.

Grains and grain products—amaranth, barley, biscuits, bran-oat, wheat, bread, corn, corn cakes, cornstarch, flour-buckwheat, hemp, kamut, potato, rice, rye, spelt, wheat, macaroni, noodles, oatmeal, pasta, quinoa, rice cakes, rolled oats, spaghetti, wheat germ.

Dairy foods—cheese yellow–cow, cheese yellow–sheep, cheese–goat, cream, ghee, ice cream, milk, yoghurt–commercial.

Vegetarian protein—adzuki beans, baked beans, black beans, bottolli beans, cashew nuts, cashew butter, chick peas, cannelloni beans, green peas, kidney beans, lentils, lima beans, macadamia nuts, navy beans, peanuts, peanut butter, pecans, pinto beans, pistachio nuts, red beans, soy beans, split peas, walnuts, white beans.

Other—artificial sweeteners, aspirin, aspartame, black pepper, caffeine, catsup, chemical drugs, corn syrup, fast foods, herbicides, honey (pasteurized), jam, jelly, medical drugs, maple syrup (processed), mayonnaise, mustard, pesticides, powdered soups, sugar and all foods with sugar added, tinned foods, tomato sauce, tobacco, vinegar.

The chart is to record your pH levels daily. It would be best to photocopy this page.

pH Chart								
	Rising	pH		Mid Morn	pH		Bed Time	pH
Date Time			Date Time			Date Time		
Date Time			Date Time			Date Time		
Date Time			Date Time			Date Time		
Date Time			Date Time			Date Time		
Date Time			Date Time			Date Time		
Date Time			Date Time			Date Time		
Date Time			Date Time			Date Time		

WATER

*J*ust how beneficial is water?

and

How much do we need?

Eighty Percent of the Human body is water:

- the brain has 85%,

- muscles have 75%,

- kidneys have 82%

- bones have 22%

- blood has 90%,

Your body needs good, clean water to survive.

*H*uman beings can go without food for several days, but not water! The body needs fluid for hydration of glands and organs. Water cleanses the body, eliminating accumulated toxins. It is needed for digestive juices and the production of saliva. Most importantly, water is needed to transport waste from the digestive system. Water also carries nutrients to the cells and is needed to help create blood plasma.

Water is essential to health. 'Good clean' water is essential to good health. We lose about two and a half litres of water a day just by breathing, perspiration and elimination. As we exhale, vapor is eliminated from the body, cleansing the bronchial system. When we perspire, fluid is also lost, and so too, of course, when eliminating waste, particularly urine, more fluid is lost from the body. Elimination of fluid is going on all the time at a considerable rate. The body cannot replace water without 'your' help; you must give your body the water it needs.

Physical problems caused by lack of water are many. The most common ones are constipation, headaches, fatigue, back problems, arthritis, cellulite and general discomfort. People could eliminate physical problems just by drinking more water.

Keep in mind that insufficient water ages the body and increases the risk of disease.

'Every function of the body is monitored and connected to the efficient flow of water to and from the body. 'Water distribution' is the only way of making sure you receive, not only an adequate amount of water you need, but its transported elements: hormones, chemical messages and nutrients. These valuable elements need to reach the vital organs to sustain life. Every organ that produces a substance to be made available to the rest of the body, will only monitor its own rate of production and release these vital elements into the 'flowing water' for distribution around the body according to constantly changing quotas set by the brain. Once the water itself reaches 'drier' areas of the body, it also exercises it's many other most vital, physical and chemical, regulatory actions. Taking this transportation system into consideration, water intake and its priority distribution purposes are of paramount importance to human survival and good health. The regulating neurotransmitter systems (histamine and its subordinate agents) become increasingly active during the regulation of water requirements of the body. Their actions should not be continuously blocked by the use of medications or toxins. Their purpose should be understood and satisfied by simply drinking more water'. (From scientific analysis — Your Body's Many Cries for Water — Batmanghelidj MD. F)

Caffeine, alcohol, and sugary foods cause dehydration. If your body is already struggling to survive disease, you are not helping it to recover if you are dehydrated. Drinking sufficient water, organic green tea, white tea, and organic herbal teas will set you on a new path to health and vitality.

You require at least two to three litres of water a day to remain hydrated. You will need more than that if you work out in the open particularly in heat, in summer, and in countries where the weather is hot and humid. If you are a gym-junkie, you may also need more than two litres a day to rehydrate muscle. Men find it more difficult to consume more than two litres of water if they have prostate problems; this varies from one man to the next, and the amount of activity he does. The best approach is to gradually increase the amount of water drunk over a period of weeks. This allows the body to adjust to the larger volume. The average person needs to drink no less than two litres a day, especially those on a cleansing program. The required amount will vary with body weight: the heavier you are, the more water you need each day.

Some people are horrified at the prospect of drinking so much water in a day; they feel they cannot do it. I hear complaints from people that when they drink a lot of water, they spend most of their time in the toilet. This alone puts them off drinking so much water. On the other hand, when the body is dehydrated, the result is like the effects of a drought on the land. When the drought breaks, the water will at first, run off the soil, and this can cause flooding. The same principle applies to the body. At first it floods; then, when the body gets used to the volume it is receiving, trips to the toilet will become less frequent. Water is now being absorbed into the system, much like soaking into the soil.

Persevere with your additional fluid intake and do not subject your body to dehydration again. It may take a few days or as much as three weeks for your body to adjust to the increase of fluid. Most individuals live their lives in a dehydrated condition. It is important to drink water not only when you are thirsty, but also when you are not. By the time you are thirsty, dehydration has already set in, and the body is crying out for help. Prevention is always better than cure!

A good way to keep up your intake of water is to distribute your daily quantity into bottles. Two to three glasses twenty minutes before breakfast. This includes your morning juice of half a lemon and warm water. Water and other liquids, should be consumed, not less than one and a half hours after food and at least twenty minutes before food. Drink water between meals not with meals. Drinking with food lessens the absorption of nutrients, and dilutes components in your digestive system. Digestion starts in the mouth. Drinking just before eating upsets the digestion and washes away digestive juices in the mouth. If you take in enough water before, and at appropriate times after a meal, your body will love you for it, and you will have more vitality.

Water filters and bottled water

In most countries, you need to drink filtered, bottled water. Alternatively you can install a water filter for your kitchen and bathroom. Beware of the water supplied to your home. Beware of the quality of the water you buy and the type of filter you install. There are many water filters on the market. Some do not work well; others are limited in their effectiveness. There are however a few really great water filters. The best type of water filter will be either a reverse osmosis or a water alkaliser.

A water alkalizer is a device using ionization to create separated alkaline water.

Your water filter needs to filter out bacteria, inorganic chemicals, lead, organic chemicals, particulate, pesticides, trihalomethanes, volatile organic chemicals, detergents, asbestos, viruses, and pollens.

The are two water filters I am aware of that are good quality, and worth the investment. One is the AlkaWay & the other is the Kangen. Both supply good quality alkaline water.

Do your homework and compare what is available before installing a filter in your home or your mobile home. Make sure that replacement components are available. You can also Google 'best water filters.' The result of this search will include technical information to help you select a water filter. Most importantly, make sure that the water filter you select produces water that is alkaline.

The body is like a sponge, it soaks up everything it receives. Be cautious about the water you use for any purpose, at home, on holidays, or at your place of work or recreation. Flukes and parasites can be found breeding in water that is impure and can infest the intestines causing inflammation and a type of gastroenteritis called Giardiasis or Giardia.

Parasite infestation can be related to cancer and being aware of the intestinal flukes and parasites in drinking water and in the washing and preparation of food is essential.

Bottled Water

Many companies supplying bottled water have jumped onto the band wagon. The quality of their product is suspect. Read the ingredients on the bottle. Make sure it has no additives or chemicals and that the product originates from a recognized, tested, organic source, bottled in regulated, hygienic conditions and preferably certified organic by the regulated authorities in the country of origin. Google search to find a good quality water, it is worth the effort.

WHY ORGANIC?

As well as ridding yourself of caffeine, sugar, drugs etc,
one of the most important things to do
is to eliminate toxic poisons.

Your body absorbs these in three ways: by ingestion, by applying them to your body or by breathing them in.

You may think eliminating toxins is impossible. I agree it is impossible to live a life of perfect harmony, especially in regard to the air we breathe unless, of course, you live in an area that is pollution free. But we can of course start with the other two vectors: what we ingest, and what we apply to our bodies.

I have already discussed eating 80% raw, 20% cooked; this is imperative if you wish to become and remain cancer free. What is just as important; is to get maximum nutrition from organic in-season fruit, vegetables, proteins and whole foods.

With the relaxation of import requirements, it is easier to import foods from overseas. In many countries throughout the world fruit and vegetables are irradiated before reaching the shelves of your local supermarket. We do not know how long the food has been stored, or where, and so there is no guarantee of freshness. Organic fresh foods contain more nutrients than food grown on land dosed with artificial fertilizers. Fruit and vegetables grown artificially have higher water content. Therefore nutrients in these fruit and vegetables are diluted.

Organic food contains fewer toxins and more nutrients, such as minerals and, vitamin C. More protective antioxidants produce more naturally occurring phyto-nutrients. They make a huge difference to our overall health and longevity. They are also essential for the prevention and cure of cancer and many other diseases. It is much safer to consume foods that are free of pesticide residues. Such residues stay in our fat cells and organs, and accumulate over time. There are up to seven pesticides used in the cultivation of mass-produced fruit and vegetables. This creates a cocktail of residues, which some researchers suggest, may be a hundred times more toxic than the individual compounds.

How does organic farming produce healthier food?

Organic farming nurtures the soil. *A gram of soil contains millions of micro organisms too small to see, and some of them are known to work with plants to help provide more nutrients. Research has shown that organically managed soil receiving compost and manure can have up to 85% more healthy soil life than if it is bombarded with chemical fertilizers and pesticides.*

Organic farming returns nutrients to the soil. *Plants remove up to 60 minerals from the soil, but non organic farmers usually replace only those necessary for plant growth — nitrogen, phosphorus and potassium. Over time this can lead to depletion of all the other minerals. Organic farmers use manures and composts containing a wide variety of minerals, so that deficiencies are less likely to develop.*

Organic farming rotates crops. *Growing the same crops each year in the same soil can lead to depletion of the nutrients used by that crop. Organic farmers rotate their crops and include "green manures" in the rotation — crops that fix nitrogen from the air into the soil, allow the soil to rest, and at the end of the season are ploughed in. All this helps prevent the soil from becoming minerally depleted, so it can go on producing healthy crops.*

Organic food contains fewer additives. *While food manufacturers can use up to 500 additives, organic food processors are prohibited from using a host of ingredients which researchers say are harmful to our health.'* (Australian Certified Organics Pty Ltd Newsletter)

Wonderful in-season produce can be bought at farmers markets, as well as at organic health food stores. Organic fresh food is usually cheaper at farmer's markets. Some vendors do not have certification from the governing organization that validates the product being organic. Their certification may be pending. Do not hesitate to ask the vendors about their products and how they are grown. Once you get to know them personally, you will know if they are genuine. But you are on safer ground if you stick with products that are organically certified and approved by the appropriate authorities. Seeking and acquiring certification is your guarantee that the vendor is serious about supplying good quality organic food.

I recommend the annual **'Clean Food Organic'**; is a complete guide to farmer's markets and organic shopping and how to access organic products in many countries. It covers food, household items, body care products and cosmetics. It also includes interesting articles and a guide to organic cafés and restaurants. You will also find directions for shopping on the internet. I can confidently recommend this book to everyone who is serious about good quality foodstuffs. It will show you how easy it is to buy organic. Their website is www.cleanfood.com — or email editor@cleanfood.com.

If you can grow some of your own food, this not only saves money, it brings you closer to nature. I live in an apartment, and grow some of my own organic herbs, tomatoes, strawberries and lettuce. I grow them in pots on the balcony. The herbs give off a beautiful aroma, as do the tomatoes. I love going out to pick a few leaves off my lettuce and herbs when preparing a salad. There is something special about being able to do this and contribute in a real way toward my own good health practices. There are many varieties of plants you can grow in pots. So why not make your garden edible? In the sub tropics or if you have a hot house in countries where the weather is cooler, lemons, which are a very important part of your regime, can be grown in pots. Give it a go, and make your own edible garden project part of your recovery program. Remember to start with bio soil, not the average supermarket kind that is laden with artificial chemicals.

Last but not least, organic farming protects the environment and the quality of the land. This will allow future generations to enjoy a healthy lifestyle. It is our responsibility to support environmental changes, so that future generations do not suffer disease as we do, through pollution of the land and environment.

Certified organic food can be more expensive in the first place. But in the long run it will prove to be more economical than conventional supermarket products. The cost of poor diets to health care alone is staggering. What is even more staggering is the number of advertising dollars spent on enticing you to buy mass-produced rubbish. Manufacturers try to convince you their processed food is good for you. Why are government authorities not protecting us from these deceptions? Processed food manufacturers are only required to list the ingredients. This is not enough. People believe advertising hype. I have heard people say, 'if it is advertised on television it must be good for you'. This statement shows how far people have been deceived.

If you want to become and stay cancer free you need to change the food you ingest, and the substances you put on your body. The following extract comes from 'Clean Food Organic' 2007, p13: "The conventional foods you must avoid". This article is well worthwhile reading, and most helpful to those who find it difficult to acquire certified organic foods.

The conventional foods you must avoid

What non-organic fresh food items consistently have the highest concentrations of pesticide residues?

Sometimes even the most prudent organic consumer may be faced with the dilemma of having to purchase regular conventional produce. Shopping out of season or away from your usual organic retailer can lead to a situation where there is no alternative. But how do you know which foods were grown with the least pesticides, and will washing or peeling them before use help reduce your exposure in any way?

Scientists from the Environmental Working Group (EWG) the USA's leading exponent of chemical related health issues, tested 43 popular conventional fruits and vegetables looking for traces of pesticide residue. They found soft skinned produce absorbs more pesticides than those with thicker skins, plus produce grown close to the ground tended to pick up more pesticides. They then compiled a list of the 12 worst offenders, nicknamed 'The Dirty Dozen'.

According to EWG spokesperson, Richard Wiles 'These (Dirty Dozen) are some of the most contaminated with pesticides, where you should buy organic.' His biggest concern though is for parents. 'Studies indicate children may be more vulnerable to toxins in pesticides. They're smaller and they eat more food relative to their size so they get a bigger dose of pesticides.' said Wiles. Interestingly, washing and peeling did not make much of a difference. All the foods in the study were thoroughly washed before testing.'

The Worst Offenders	Better Choice (but still grown with pesticides)
1. Peaches	1. Onions
2. Apples	2. Avocado
3. Capsicum	3. Sweet Corn (frozen)
4. Celery	4. Pineapple
5. Nectarines	5. Mango
6. Strawberries	6. Asparagus
7. Cherries	7. Sweet Peas (frozen)
8. Pears	8. Kiwi Fruit
9. Grapes	9. Bananas
10. Spinach	10. Cabbage
11. Lettuce	11. Broccoli
12. Potatoes	12. Papaya

Know what is in your bathroom, kitchen and laundry

Many people do not realize that what they apply to their skin can be toxic. Personal care products can cause illnesses, particularly cancers. The few items below discuss the most commonly used chemicals in products and their effects. Most of the information comes from 'The Chemical Maze Shopping Companion — Your Guide to Food Additives and Cosmetic Ingredients ' written by Bill Statham, a book I highly recommend and that fits easily into your handbag or pocket. With this on hand you can be an informed shopper, no longer in the dark about what chemicals are harmful to you and what chemicals are used in the products you buy. 'The Chemical Maze Shopping Companion — Your Guide to Food Additives and Cosmetic Ingredients' is essential. There are other books which are also informative, but I find that Bill Statham's book is the easiest to follow, especially because I can carry it with me. The author makes it easy to recognize additives and ingredients that cause discomfort and ill health in foods, personal care products, and cosmetics.

'Silent Killers' and 'Read the Label, Know the Risks' both written by P. M. Taubert are two other books for your bookshelf and are also very informative.

ITEM 1—Sodium Lauryl sulphate (SLS) also known as Sodium Laureth sulfate

A foaming agent used in shampoos, hair conditioners, detergents, cake mixes, marshmallows, dried egg products, bubble bath, liquid hand and body wash, moisturisers, toothpaste, cosmetics, industrial cleaning products, degreasing agents, car wash detergent and antibiotic tablets.

Potential Side Effects and Health Risks: Cataracts, improper eye development in infants and children, corneal damage, skin cancer, liver toxicity and liver cancer, dermatitis, mouth ulcers, impaired hair growth and, corrosion of hair follicles. It may be contaminated with carcinogen 1, 4–Dioxane. This additive is on the National Institute of Health (NIH) Hazard List as *Teratogen.

SLS is used in many so-called 'natural products'. Do not trust the word 'natural' on a label. Do not accept the description and presume that the product is good for you. Read the label in full. If it is so small you need a magnifying glass to read it, leave the product on the shelf and find something similar with a label you can read. Then you will know if that product is safe.

Stop for a moment and consider that SLS is a poison. It is in many of the products used by most people, often first thing in the morning, even before breakfast. What a way to start your day!

ITEM 2—Monosodium l-glutamate also know as MSG or 621, E621

MSG is a flavour enhancer. It is found in many takeaway foods, packet soups, soy sauce, flavoured noodles, meats, malt extract, quick soup, pickles, sauce, gelatin, maltodextrin. It is also an ingredient in soaps, shampoos, cosmetics and hair conditioners, where it is a hidden additive.

Potential Side Effects and Health Risks: Asthma, hyperactivity, depression, irritability, mood changes, chest pain, nausea, numbness, migraine, headaches, infertility, convulsions, abdominal discomfort. MSG is also on the NIH Hazard List as *Teratogen.

* Teratogen: *"An agent that can disturb the development of an embryo or fetus causing birth defects".* www.medterms.com

ITEM 3—Talc – 553 E553b

Talc is a naturally occurring mineral. It is not classified as food grade by the Food and Drug Administration (FDA). It is powdered soapstone used as a base in baby powder, bath powder, face powder, and as filler in creams. Some sources of talc are contaminated with asbestos. Talc is also used as an anti-caking agent for confectionery, polished rice, chocolate, chewing gum and in the manufacture of condoms.

Potential Side Effects and Health Risks: Cancer (Stomach and Ovarian), respiratory problems, irritation to the eyes and a cause of fibrotic pneumoconiosis, infertility and Non-Hodgkin's Lymphoma.

ITEM 4—Aluminium

Used in antiperspirants, face powders and other cosmetics, toothpaste, astringents, antiseptics, detergents, and aspirin. Cooking pots, and drink cans are made from aluminum. It is also employed as surface colouring in some foods.

Potential Side Effects and Health Risks: Osteoporosis, cancer, dementia, Alzheimer's disease, Parkinson type illnesses, kidney and lung disorders, irritability, infection of the skin and hair follicles and extremely toxic to the body.

ITEM 5 – Sulphur dioxide (220, E220)

Sulphur dioxide is a preservative used in commercial, non-organic, dried fruit, beer, fruit juice, gelatin, wine, soft drinks, cordial, jam, dairy products, potato products, soup, and glue. It is also used as a disinfectant in breweries and food factories.

Potential Side Effects and Health Risks: Asthma, hyperactivity, headache, backache, gastric irritation, liver toxicity, bronchitis, nausea. It destroys vitamin A in food.

There are of course, many, many more additives. No wonder they require a book on their own. It is tragic that so many dangerous, toxic poisons are permitted by law to be included in everyday cleaning and personal care items. Is it any wonder so many people have health issues and cancer? You can invest in your health and safety by acquiring either the 'The Chemical Maze' book or 'Silent Killers'. In the meantime, make a note of additive numbers you find so you can avoid them.

Your own chemical free environment

Always use certified organic products in your home, or products that are at least chemical-free. You need to take responsibility for yourself and the members of your family. Changing over to certified organics is only the first step to improving your health and combating disease. Make loud and clear complaints to the multi-nationals who are poisoning your food, your home, and personal care products. Buy only organic and chemical-free items. The more people who protest through their shopping habits, the quicker growers, manufacturers and governments will take notice.

There are today, many excellent chemical-free personal products for your face, hair and nails. There are certified organic products that are not expensive or dangerous to health. I personally have not, knowingly, used any chemicals on my body for many years.

A website that is worth visiting especially if you are not in an area where you can buy organic and chemical free products is www.iherb.com. The sell nutritional supplements, personal care products for the whole family, environmentally friendly laundry products, skin care products, makeup, and a large variety of food products. They will ship internationally.

Such businesses are to be found throughout the world. Use an internet search engine to find them.

Personal care products are very personal and we all like different things. The list that begins on the following page contains some of my own favourite choices. These are products I love and find excellent for not only my skin and body. You can be sure they do not contain poisons. My choice of household products is also included.

y List

Toothpaste

Gano Fresh Ganoderma Toothpaste

To buy, go to resources.

Mouth Wash

Miessence Organic Freshening Mouth Wash

Buy online www.miessence.com or health food stores.

Soap, Bath and Shower washes

Lavera Organic Skincare & Cosmetics for men, women and children

Buy online or to find your nearest stockist. www.lavera.com

Rich Hippie Organic Body & Bath

Buy online www.rich-hippie.com

Aubrey Organics Bar Soap

Buy online www.iherb.com or from health food stores and/or pharmacies.

Shampoo and Conditioner

Lavera Organic Skincare & Cosmetics for men, women and children

Buy online or find your nearest stockist. www.lavera.com

Miessence Organic Shampoo & Conditioner

Buy online www.miessence.com or health food stores.

Insect Repellent

Miessence Organic Buzz Free Zone Personal Spray

Buy online www.miessence.com or health food stores.

Badger Company Anti-Bug Balm

Buy online www.iherb.com or health food stores.

Lavera Organic Skincare & Cosmetics for men, women and children

Buy online or find your nearest stockist. www.lavera.com

Rich Hippie Organic Perfumes

Buy online www.rich-hippie.com or health food stores

Carmaje Organics

Buy online or to find your nearest stockist. www.carmaje.com.au

Miessence Organic Skin Care

Buy online www.miessence.com or health food stores.

Sunscreen, Lip Balm

Lavera Organic Skincare & Cosmetics

Buy online or find your nearest stockist. www.lavera.com

Soleo Organics

Buy online www.iherb.com or selected health food stores/pharmacies.

Sunless Tanning

Lavera Organic Skincare & Cosmetics

Buy online or find your nearest stockist. www.lavera.com

Lip Balm

Coco Lip Balm

Buy online or to find your nearest stockist. www.thaiorganiclife.com

Lavera Organics Skincare & Cosmetics

Buy online or to find your nearest stockist. www.lavera.com

Deodorant

Crystal Body Deodorant

Buy online at www.iherb.com or at health food stores, and pharmacies.

Sacred Kingdom Essences

Buy online www.sacredkingdomessences.com

Pranadevi

Buy online www.pranadevi.net

Donna Louise Spiritual Sprays and Products

Buy online or to find your nearest stockist. www.donnalouise.com.au

Essential Oils

Perfect Potions

Buy online or to find your nearest stockist. www.perfectpotions.com

Makeup inclusive of Foundation, Eye Makeup, Lipstick etc.

Lavera Organic Skincare & Cosmetics

Buy online or find your nearest stockist. www.lavera.com

Hair Dyes

Aubrey Organic Color Me Natural

Buy online. www.iherb.com or health food stores.

Herbatint

To find your nearest stockist. www.herbatint.com

Hair Spray

Lavera Organic Skincare & Cosmetics

Buy online or to find your nearest stockist www.lavera.com

Nail Polish and Remover

Suncoat Products

Buy online or to find your nearest stockist. www.suncoatproducts.com

Ecover

To find your nearest stockist or buy online go to www.ecover.com

Ecostore

To find your nearest stockist or to buy online go to www.ecostore.com

Laundry Powder

Ecover

To find your nearest stockist or buy online go to www.ecover.com

Ecostore Laundry Powder

Buy online or to find your nearest stockist. www.ecostore.com

57

From Cancer to Wellness — the forgotten secrets

Notes

Chapter One

DIGESTION AND THE ABSORPTION OF NUTRIENTS

*E*ating smaller meals, in a relaxed environment aids digestion.

"In general, mankind since the improvement of cookery eats twice as much as nature requires."

Benjamin Franklin.

*T*he digestive system is overstressed by eating too much, or eating too fast. Generally less is usually best. Food should be chewed and eaten in a relaxed way. People tend to have a fast moving lifestyle. They always seem to be in a hurry, and often forget to sit quietly and eat their meals in comfort and with pleasure. As a result many of us do not digest our food properly. While we are 'on the run' valuable nutrients are not being absorbed into our system from the food we have eaten.

Have you ever considered the importance of mealtimes? Who you share a meal with? Where you eat and how? Also, how much time have you given yourself to enjoy your meal? Meal-times need to be special pleasant occasions, not stressful or chaotic. Eating 'on the run' or when we are stressed or hurried, is not good for the digestion. Also, we make bad food choices when we do not allow time for meals. People tend to grab what is easily available, what is easy to get, or cheap to buy. They do not think about the harm that food will do to their body.

The old parental instruction "Chew your food slowly" remains as valid today as it ever was. Chewing slowly aids digestion and makes the transfer of food into your system as smooth as possible. It is vital if you want to get well and stay well. As a guide each mouthful of food should be chewed thirty times and mixed with saliva to activate liver secretions. To focus on this aspect of your meal, you need to slow down and think about what you are doing. This attitude alone is helpful to digestion. When eating is a pleasurable experience, neurotransmitters such as serotonin and noradrenalin are released. This enhances our feeling of well-being, and helps us become more alert. The opposite happens after a hurried, health-destroying meal; we feel weighed down by the meal.

Always sit at a table away from your work environment to eat a meal. Leave your work on your desk, or wherever it may be, and give yourself a well-deserved break! Light candles at dinner, whenever possible, to create an atmosphere of relaxation and pleasure, even when eating alone. Surround yourself with pleasant sounds and aromas and have your meals with people who are caring, fun, and pleasant to be with. Bless the food and be thankful for what you are about to eat and thank those who prepared it for you.

Here is some logical, sensible advice:

"Diet has the distinction of being the only major determinant of health that is completely under our control. You have the final say over what does and does not go into your mouth and stomach. You cannot always control the other determinants of health, such as quality of the air you breathe, the noise you are subject to or the emotional climate of your surroundings, but you can control what you eat. It is a shame to squander such a good opportunity to influence your health" (Weil in Carper, 1998, pp 17–18 in Food as Medicine Subject Guide pp1.4 M. Blondel and Australian College of Natural Medicine)

Some foods go through the digestive system faster than others. Fruit for instance, is digested faster than protein; so fruit needs to be eaten first. Have you ever had an evening meal, followed by fruit salad and then found you felt bloated and full of gas from the meal? Protein and other cooked vegetables take longer to digest so the fruit seems to sits on top of the other food and ferments.

It is important to pay attention to how you combine foods in a meal. But it is equally important to take them in the right sequence. Foods, such as the tomato, (which is a fruit) combine well with non-starchy vegetables and nuts and avocado. It is important to know about good and bad food combinations. Commit the basic facts to memory. This will assist you when you are eating out. See food combining chart.

Once you remember which food combines well with other foods, you can combine ingredients in ways that make your meals not only appealing to the pallet, but also healing to your body.

Simple rules when eating:

- Avoid cold foods, as they delay digestion.

- Very hot drinks distress your stomach. It is best to drink liquids that are neither too hot nor too cold.

- Black pepper and chilli peppers eat away the stomach lining, except for cayenne pepper which has healing properties and works as a catalyst for other herbs to heal faster.

- Soda and baking powders derange food chemistry and also eat away the stomach lining.

- Avoid fried, spicy and sugary foods as they cause stomach distress.

- Avoid vinegar and alcohol, along with other fermented foods, as they set in motion fermentation in the stomach. The exception to this rule is apple cider vinegar, which aids digestion when taken with warm water 20 minutes before a meal.

- Processed heated oil and fats slow down digestion.

- Eating between meals and overeating both retard digestion. Leave at least four to five hours between meals.

- Drinking at mealtimes and eating watery food slow down digestion by diluting digestive juices in the stomach. Never drink with meals. The rule is: do not eat food earlier than twenty minutes after drinking and do not drink for two hours after eating.

- Food needs to be chewed slowly and mixed with saliva to activate liver secretions.

- Digestion starts in the mouth; drinking just before eating inhibits this important stage.

- Avoid foods you are allergic to; as they will interfere with digestion and absorption of nutrients, not to mention the bad effect on your immune system.

- Combine foods that complement each other. See food combining chart in the following pages.

- Food that digests faster than other foods, such as fruit and vegetables should to be eaten first.

- Avoid too much cooked food in the evening; this is a time to eat light meals.

*E*at breakfast like
a King,

*E*at lunch like a Prince,
and

*D*ine in the evening
like a Pauper.

Old German Proverb

The food combining chart on these two pages is a guide to the way each food group suits others in order to facilitate the breakdown of foods in the digestive system through the action of digestive enzymes.

SWEET FRUIT

All dried fruits, bananas, custard apples, dates, figs, and persimmon

> *Combine well with* sub-acid fruits, acid fruits, grains & grain products, dairy products

SUB ACID FRUIT

Apples, apricots, avocado, blackberries, blueberries, cherries, grapes, guava, lychee, mangos, nectarines, olives, papaya, peaches, pears, quince, raspberries

> *Combine well with* sweet fruit, acid fruit, vegetables, grains and grain products, nuts, seeds, animal products, dairy products

ACID FRUIT

Currants, grapefruit, kiwi fruit, kumquats, lemons, limes, loganberries, oranges, passion fruit, pineapples, plums, strawberries, tangerines, tomatoes

> *Combine well with* sub acid fruit, sweet fruit, vegetables, grain and grain products, legumes, nuts, seeds, animal products, dairy products

MELONS TO BE EATEN ALONE

Casaba, honeydew, rock melon, watermelon, other melons

NON STARCH VEGETABLES

Asparagus, broccoli, brussels sprouts, cabbage, capsicum, cauliflower, celery, choko, cucumber, egg plant, kohlrabi, leek, lettuce, onion, parsley, silver beet, spinach, sprouts, squash, zucchini

> *Combine well with* most foods except melons and sweet fruit

STARCH VEGETABLES

Artichoke, beetroot, carrot, parsnip, potato, pumpkin, radish, sweet potato, turnip

> *Combine well with* non starch vegetables, animal products, and dairy products

ANIMAL PRODUCTS

Bacon, beef, chicken, clams, crab, crayfish, crustaceans, duck, eggs, fish, goose, lamb, lobster, oysters pork, quail, rabbit, veal

> *Combine well with* sub acid fruit, acid fruit, non starch vegetables, starch vegetables, grains and grain products, dairy products

NUTS & SEEDS

Alfalfa, almonds, brazil, cashews, chestnuts, coconuts, hazel, macadamia, pecan, pistachio, pumpkin seeds, sesame seeds, sunflower seeds, walnuts

> *Combine well with* sub acid fruits, acid fruit, non starch vegetables, grain and grain products, and dairy products

LEGUMES

Adzuki beans, baked beans, black-eye peas & beans, broad beans, carob beans, chickpeas, falafel, hyacinth peas, kidney beans, lentils, lima beans, mung beans, peanuts, peas, runner beans, soya beans

> *Combine well with* acid fruits, non starch vegetables, starch vegetables, grains & grain products, and dairy products

DAIRY & OTHER PRODUCE

Butter, cheese, chocolate, cream, ice-cream, milk, mayonnaise, yoghurt

> *Combine with* all food groups with the exception of melons

GRAIN & GRAIN PRODUCTS

Barley, biscuits, bread, bulgur, cakes, corn-maize, millet, oats, pasta, pastry, pizza, rice, rye, sorghum, wheat

> *Combine well with* sweet fruit, sub-acid fruit, acid fruit, non starch vegetables, legumes, nuts, seeds, animal products and dairy products

CANDIDA AND THE PARASITE CONNECTION

In order for the body to heal, it must be able to
absorb all the nutrients that you are now going to give it.

The first thing to do is to improve your digestive system and enhance your immune system. There are many reasons why your digestive system might not be functioning properly. But our purpose here is to look forward and heal, not to look back and blame.

You may have experienced an increase in digestive problems over the years. The most common reasons are — a diet deficient in proper nutrients, impure water, coupled with the overuse of antibiotics, oral contraceptives, corticosteroid drugs, and other medications.

We are seeing more people suffering from Crohn's disease, irritable bowel syndrome, leaky gut, diverticulitis, celiac disease, indigestion, reflux, allergies, asthma and constipation. Parasites and other harmful organisms that affect the immune system are on the increase. The most common of these is Candida Albicans. All this shows the need for better nutrition through a healthy diet.

It is crucial to increase and maintain bacteria levels, eliminate any yeast infection and parasite infestation, thus help rid the body of cancer.

Someone said to me: "People do not die of cancer, they die of malnutrition". I believe this is true. A body that is not getting the right nutrition cannot be expected to heal itself and fight off disease.

Plenty of organic raw foods will keep the bowel free from constipation. The body has to balance bacteria levels, combat yeast infection and eliminate parasites. People do not realize that the human body is a perfect place for parasites. They accept that children become infested with parasites and will give their children a dose of medication. But once past the toddler stage, parasite prevention and eradication is stopped. It is quite unusual for an adult to be treated.

Attention to parasite infestation is no less important for adults. Follow the protocols described below to rid your body of parasites. However, you will also need to find out if you have candida infection.

Candida

Candida, or Candida Albicans, to give it its full name, is an overgrowth of a single cell yeast-like fungus. This fungus is referred to in Eastern cultures as a dampness affecting various parts of the body most commonly the gastrointestinal tract and the vagina. The digestive system and metabolism is compromised by the often prolific growth in the body by this yeast. Those having a weakened immune system almost always have high levels of candida, especially those suffering from advanced cancer, HIV and AIDS. In extreme cases the infection will travel through the bloodstream and affect every organ of the body.

People suffering from candida become very sensitive to certain foods. They find some smells intolerable, especially petrol, cigarettes, exhaust fumes, perfumes, cleaning products, and rubber.

Test yourself for candida without a visit to the doctor or the naturopath. Proceed as follows:

1. Place a glass of water on your bedside table or on your bathroom cabinet before going to bed.

2. First thing in the morning, spit into the water. Do not eat or drink anything before this (this is important).

3. Let the saliva sit in the water for about 30 minutes but no more than an hour before testing.

4. Check the water to see if it is clear. If you see strands of saliva (like legs) floating in the water or cloudy saliva that has sunk to the bottom of the glass, or floating in the water, then you have candida.

If you have candida, it will need to be cleared up immediately. The removal of parasites from your system is also imperative if you want to absorb nutrients from your food. For cancer sufferers, it is usually the fluke worm that is the problem.

This is the opinion of Dr Hulda Regehr Clark, author of 'The Cure for All Cancers', 'The Cure for All Diseases' and 'The Cure for All Advanced Cancers'.

You will definitely have parasites if you have cancer or candida. Remember:

- The candida yeast feeds off sugar.
- Your body's pH balance is important for friendly bacteria such as lactobacilli to thrive. These are needed to metabolise sugars properly.

Weeks 1 to 4

(This chapter has been set out for you to eradicate both parasites and candida. Many of the following foods and beverages you will be avoiding permanently.):

Foods to avoid

- ✗ Remove all foods that contain sugar, honey, malt etc. and yeast from your diet; this includes yeasted breads, cakes, buns, rolls, pastries, crackers (unless sugar and yeast free), enriched flour, anything fried in breadcrumbs, truffles and chocolate.

- ✗ Eat no fruit, including sweet fruits, dried fruits, and acid fruits. Do this only for four weeks.

- ✗ All yeast spreads. (Vegemite, Marmite etc.)

- ✗ Black tea and herbal teas. The two exceptions are Pau D'Arco tea, known for its anti fungal properties (two to three cups per day is sufficient), and Black Walnut Herbal Tea, which is helpful for the elimination of parasites.

- ✗ Coffee.

- ✗ Mushrooms.

- ✗ Dairy milk — (you can replace it with coconut milk, oat milk or rice milk). Make sure they are sugar and malt free.

- ✗ Cheese.

- ✗ Alcohol, soft drinks, citrus drinks frozen or canned, fermented foods such as soy, vinegar, soy sauce, honey, peanut butter, pickles, stock and soup cubes, alfalfa sprouts, and vitamin B tablets that contain yeast,

- ✗ Enriched flour or anything made from 'baker's flour' which contains yeast and chemical improvers.

Nutrients and foods to take

✔ Multi-strain probiotic. Use a dairy free formula.

✔ Paracea to remove parasites and worms, Paracea also helps digestive function and fights candida.

✔ Kolorex herbal antifungal formula.

✔ Garlic oil which has a yeast killing effect in the intestines.

✔ Bromelain between meals facilitates the digestion of dietary protein (the best formula to purchase is Nutrition Diagnostics Bio-zyme Formula).

✔ Co-Enzyme Q10 daily.

✔ A diet high in fibre. Eat lots of fresh vegetables, yeast free grains such as brown rice, millet, and non fermented vegetarian protein.

✔ Eat live cultured yoghurts that are sugar and juice free.

✔ Replace your toothbrush every two weeks or disinfect with either a solution of water and citric seed acid or apple cider vinegar.

I have included the active ingredients in all nutritional supplementation charts. It will enable you to buy similar products if the brands nominated are not available to you. All products I have recommended contain quality ingredients. Most are provided by naturopaths or doctors committed to advancing complementary medicine. This type of practitioner will have a degree in Nutritional Medicine. Although the nutritional supplements recommended in this handbook will not be harmful to you, it is however recommended that you seek professional advice from your health care practitioner. He or she will check the dosages and may recommend an alternative product.

If you live in an area where you are unable to buy what you need or you do not have a reliable holistic health care pracitioner you can go to my site www. cancertowellness. Click on Doctors & Support. This will lead you to Jack at the Broadbeach Compound Pharmacy - you will need then click on www.ewell.com. and follow the prompts. You can also email them for more information info@ ewell.com.au or phone Jack on +61 7 56770562. This pharmacy will send orders wordwide.

Nutritional Supplements

SUPPLEMENT AND DOSAGE	COMMENTS AND ACTIVE INGREDIENTS
Probiotics **Nutrition Care Lactobac Powder** or similar — use a non dairy formula. 5 ml level spoonful 2 times daily — 1 hour before meals.	Fights candida Infection, balances bacteria levels in the stomach. **Active Ingredients:** *Lactobacillus rhamnosus* 14.25 billion organisms, *Bifidobacterium* longum 750 million organisms.
Bioceuticals Paracea Forte or similar 2 capsules 3 times daily before meals (breakfast, lunch and dinner). *When taking Paracea or similar product it is important to take for 2 weeks, then 5 days off, then 2 weeks on again — this is to make sure any eggs that hatch are destroyed.*	Helps to maintain a healthy digestive function and rid body of parasites, worms, bacteria, and candida and gut disturbances. **Active Ingredients:** Artemisia herb (Chinese Wormwood), *Berberis vulgaris* (Barberry) stem bark, *Juglans nigra* (Black Walnut) fruit hull, Citrus x paradise (Grapefruit) fruit.
Bioceuticals Quercetin (or similar) (Includes Bromelain for improve absorption of quercetin.) 600mg twice daily between meals.	Spreads healing and helps reduce the effects of inflammation and allergic conditions together with the Bromelain to provide nutritional support. **Active Ingredients:** Quercetin, Bromelain.
Nutrition Diagnostics Bio-Zyme Formula 1 capsule to be taken 30 minutes before meals. or similar	Promotes digestion, breaks down plaque in the arteries, thins blood, and stops the growth of malignant cells in many forms of cancer. It enhances the immune system and defends against candida. **Active Ingredients:** Bromelains, Papain, Extracts equivalent to fresh: Cynara scolymus (leaf), Extracts equivalent to dry: Zingiber officinale (root), Powders, Gentiana lutea (root), Cinnamomum zeylanicum stem bark.
Kolorex from Forest Herbs 1 x Aniseed and 1 x Horopito simultaneously once a day.	A stringent anti-fungal and helps to maintain a balanced intestinal flora. **Active Ingredients:** (New Zealand Herb Horopito (Pseudowintera colorata), Aniseed.
Garlic Oil 2 capsules twice daily.	Inhibits the growth of the infecting organism. Excellent for eradicating candida, colds and bacterial infections. **Active Ingredients:** Each capsule contains fresh pure garlic oil.

SUPPLEMENT AND DOSAGE	COMMENTS AND ACTIVE INGREDIENTS
Nature's Way, Alive! Organic Vitamin C Powder 2 heaped teaspoon twice daily in 200 ml water and the juice of 1/2 a lemon. or **Nutrition Diagnostics Bio-Vitamin C Powder**	Builds up immunity and protects body tissue from any further damage by the release of toxins. **Active Ingredients:** 100% Whole Food Complex derives its entire vitamin C content from organic fruit sources, Acerola, Goji, Amla and kiwi. **Active Ingredients:** Ascorbic Acid, Lycine, Glycine, Proline, Citrus Bioflavonoids Extract, Green Tea, Catechins, Epigallochatechin 3-0 Gallate.
Bioceuticals Multi Essentials 1 tablet daily with food, due to the strength of this formulation it must be taken with food to avoid nausea. Or IntraMAX Liquid All in one dietary supplement. For further information see IntraMAX under nutritional supplements in Chapter 4.	Multi Essential Vitamins are needed for proper immune function and used in conjunction with other remedies will aid absorption of other nutrients. **Active Ingredients:** Mixed Tocopherols, Betatene, Ascorbic Acid ,Natural vitamin E (as succinate), vitamin A (as retinyl palmitate), vitamin B1 (thiamine, vitamin B2 (riboflavin), vitamin B3 (nicotinamide), vitamin B6 (pyridoxine, hydrochloride), vitaminB5 (calcium pantothenate), vitamin B12,Folic Acid, vitamin D3, vitamin K1, Calcium citrate, Manganese amino acid chelate, Zinc amino acid chelate, Copper gluconate, Selenomethionine, Magnesium Oxide, Chromium nicotinate, Biotin, Choline bitartate, Inositol, Molybdenum trioxide, Boron, Bioflavonoids. Supplies a balanced vitamin B complex with extra B12 for healthy methylation and homocysteine metabolism. Provides 2:1 ratio of Calcium to magnesium with boron, for healthy bone support.
Orthoplex Repairase 1 teaspoons twice daily	The combination of antioxidants, anti-inflammatory, is immune supportive, has antiviral activities and repairs internal and external tissue. **Active ingredients:** Quercetin, Rutin, Magnesium ascorbate, Bromelains, Zinc gluconate, Calcium pantothenate, Selenomethionine, d-alpha tocopherol succinate, retinyl palmitate.

Also helpful for fighting candida:

- **Organic Aloe Vera** has an anti fungal action. It boosts the white blood cells' ability to kill yeast cells, as well as improving overall bowel flora. Aloe Vera is also supportive when combined with the nutritional protocols in 'Program for Life', and 'Optimum Daily Program' contained in this handbook. I recommend that you use only organic Aloe Vera.

- **Slippery Elm** helps to soothe inflamed areas of the mucous lining of the stomach and bowel.

- **Vitamineral Greens** is an extremely potent and comprehensive array of nature's most nutritive and cleansing superfoods, grown and processed to maximize their benefits. It contains a full spectrum of naturally occurring, absorbable and non-toxic vitamins, minerals, all essential amino acids (protein), antioxidants, chlorophyll, soluble and insoluble fibers, thousands of phytonutrients, and a plethora of other synergistically bound, organic nutrients. It contains no synthetic or isolated nutrients (and is not excreted as expensive yellow urine or stored as toxic deposits). Vitamineral Green is actual food. Go to www.rawpower.com.

- **Coconut milk and coconut oil** help fight dangerous micro-organisms in the body. The lauric acid in coconuts is the same medium chain fatty acid (MCFA) found in mother's milk. This compound is a substance that has been shown to inactivate numerous viruses, bacteria, yeast and fungi. (See: Healthy Bites from Nutrition Diagnostics.) To review the benefits of coconut oil and its products visit www.westongprice.org. Also google www.nuicoconut.com.

  Make sure coconut milk or coconut cream is certified organic. You can water down coconut cream and milk. Store it in a glass container in the refrigerator after it has been opened.

Let thy food be thy medicine.

Hippocrates

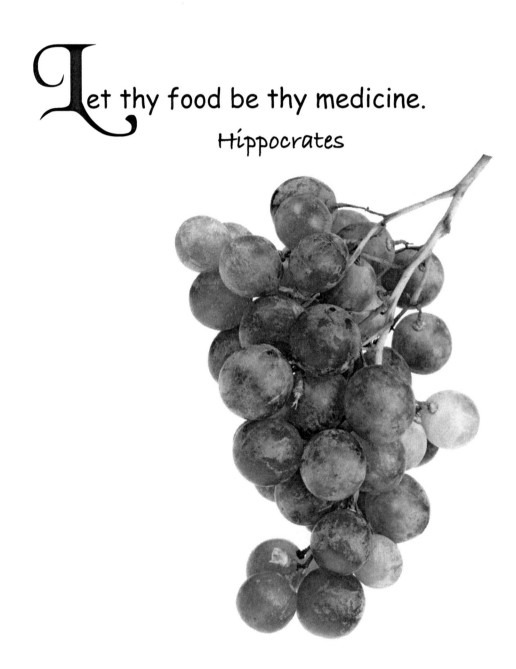

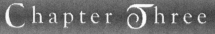

MAKING FOOD YOUR MEDICINE

The ancient physician, Hippocrates is called the "Father of Medicine"
Hippocratic medicine was humble and passive and the therapeutic approach
was based on "the healing power of nature" (Wikipedia).

Hippocrates advocated using food to heal the body.
He maintained that the body is a self-healing mechanism.

I have set out a program in this book to beat cancer. It will not suppress or manipulate your immune system in the same way as pharmaceutical drugs. Your body will receive what it needs in order to heal itself. Even though there is no such thing as a quick fix with healing; the rate of your healing will depend on your individual system, and its nutritional deficiencies. Your body will heal when given the opportunity through self nurturing. You must be prepared for it to take time to get back into shape. Natural healing is not an overnight fix and you many feel a little off colour in the first few days of starting this program because your body is ridding itself of accumulated toxins.

Healing Crisis

Healing Crisis is another way to describe the effects of detoxing. This means you may feel worse before you feel better, and before your healing happens. You may feel scared and want to quit or take a drug. **Please do not do either.** Your body is releasing toxins and poisons that must be eliminated. This is a warning to stay focused and allow the body to 'win'.

You may experience fatigue, and headaches. Urine may go dark and bowels may smell really foul. Your tongue may be coated and you might feel irritable and weak, not to mention nauseous. Brain fog may set in and diarrhoea, flu-like symptoms, and a fever. The healing crisis will pass, and beleive me it will be worth it!

To keep these symptoms to a minimum — drink plenty of water and herbal teas to help with elimination. Have colonics or enemas regularly. Stick to the regime and rest, **REST A LOT!** Give your body the time and space to start healing.

Living Valley Springs (LVS) have produced and sell a very effective herbal tea, which is designed to assist the organs eliminate at a deep tissue level. You can purchase this tea through LVS (or make it yourself) — it is called Living Valley Springs Cleanse Tea and it is a combination of chaparral, corn silk, ginger, elder flower, peppermint, red clover, and chamomile. The chart on the following two pages describes the effects of these herbs on the body.

If you are a carbohydrate addict, addicted to processed foods, particularly sugar, it will take seven to ten days to withdraw from these poisons. If you are addicted to caffeine, then it is quite common to expect headaches for up to two to four days.

Remember this quote and rely on it during your detox period:

"The body is made by design to win. Once interference has been identified and removed, the body can recover from just about anything."
(Martin, Gary, ND AFAIM, Life Style Excellence Newsletter, September–November 2007 Page 2, Living Valley Springs, Kin Kin, Australia).

"Let thy food be thy medicine"

Hippocrates

HERB	BENEFITS	COMMENTS
CHAMOMILE	Anti-inflammatory, antiseptic capabilities, stress, anxiety and nerve tonic, aids digestion, sleep tonic, muscle relaxant and antispasmodic. Used in the relief of menstrual cramps, assists in the promotion of a natural hormone — thyroxin. Chamomile is also helpful for colitis, diverticulitis, headaches, pain and fever, also improves mental alertness and is a useful mouthwash and diuretic.	Should not be taken daily over long periods of time: Not to be taken with alcohol or sedatives.
CHAPARRAL	Ability to deep cleanse into the muscle and tissue walls, is a strong antioxidant, fights free radicals and chelates heavy metals. It is said to remove residue of LSD out of the system. Anti-tumor agent, protects against cancer cells, analgesic, antiseptic, is one of the best herbal antibiotics. Has anti-HIV activity, also protects against harmful effects of radiation and sun exposure.	Taken over prolonged periods and/or in large doses can cause liver damage.
CORN SILK	Aids in kidney, bladder conditions, and helps to remove gravel from kidneys, bladder and prostate gland. Good for carpal tunnel syndrome, obesity, PMS. Used in combination with other kidney herbs to open the urinary tract and remove mucus from the urine. Is good for dropsy and edema when a weak heart is the cause. Corn Silk has anti-inflammatory benefits in connection to conditions of the urethra, bladder, prostate, and kidneys.	
ELDER FLOWER	Combats free radicals. Superior tonic and blood purifier, eases constipation, enhances immune system, lowers fever, stops glands swelling, and detoxifies the body at a cellular level. Is effective against flu viruses, stimulates circulation, relieves pain, purges the lungs, increases perspiration, soothes respiratory tract and is good for the liver, kidneys, headaches, rheumatism and epilepsy.	Not to be taken during pregnancy. Avoid the stems of this plant as they contain cyanide.
GINGER	Supports the digestive and respiratory system, fights inflammation, and stimulates circulation. Excellent agent for cleansing the bowels, kidneys and the skin. Used for such disorders as arthritis, fever, hot flushes, headaches, sore throat, car and sea sickness, morning sickness. Is a blood thinner and combines well with other herbs to enhance their effectiveness. Is a strong antioxidant and good for fighting off colds and flu.	Not recommended if taking anticoagulants or have gall stones.

HERB	BENEFITS	COMMENTS
PEPPERMINT	Acts as a muscle relaxant, particularly in the digestive tract. Increases acidity and so aids digestion. Has a slightly anesthetic effect on the mucous membranes and the gastrointestinal tract. Used in the treatments of chills, fever, colic, diarrhoea, headaches, heart trouble, heart palpitations, nausea, indigestion, irritable bowel syndrome, vomiting, poor appetite, rheumatism, spasms. A general stimulant for the whole body and strengthens the whole system.	
RED CLOVER	Works as a blood purifier, fights infections, improves circulation stimulates the secretion of bile. Has antispasmodic, and relaxing effects, soothes nerves and cleans the bronchi, is a superior cancer treatment herb — a must in any detox and healing formula. Good for HIV and AIDS symptoms.	

PROGRAM FOR LIFE

A 28 day detox,
to get your body into a state of alkalinity,
where cancer cells cannot survive.

On the next page the program begins with four transitioning in days of raw food only. This helps to clear the body of heavy solids. It also reduces the initial side effects as your body rids itself of toxins, and gently prepares your body for juicing. This is followed by a 20 days of juices and broths, together with a couple of days of solid food in the middle of each ten day section.

The program ends with four transitioning out days similar to the transitioning in days to support the body's digestive system and gently introducing you back to solid food again.

Included in the program is recommended nutritional supplements together with the suggested dosages.

You will feel great after this and your liver will love you for it. Juicing will increase your energy levels and you will feel so CLEAN inside and out. Juicing gives the body a buzz, like the buzz received from exercising; endorphins kick in, depression and all ill feeling goes and a new person is born.

Your liver will be cleansed. This is so very important because around 80–90% of the blood that leaves the stomach and intestinal tract carries nutrients to the liver where they are converted into substances the body can use. The liver metabolizes and processes carbohydrates, fats, minerals and proteins used in maintaining healthy bodily functions.

𝒰pon rising around 6.00 am (or earlier if you wish)

- Test pH level and record, clean teeth, scrape tongue, and take a shower.

30 mins later:

- 1 glass of warm (not hot) water with the juice of half a fresh lemon, together with 2 tsp vitamin C powder and 1 sachet of Percy's Powder to help alkaline your body. To this add liquid vitamins, minerals and eight drops of Cellfood or see IntraMax protocols if choosing this product in place of liquid vitamins, minerals and Cellfood.

- 2 capsules of Paracea parasite herbs or 7.5mls liquid wormwood herb mixture.

- 2 capsules Co-Enzyme Q10, 3 tbsp coconut oil, 2 Capsules EPA/DHA Omega 3, 1 tsp probiotic.

- 1 long glass of water 10 minutes later.

- Early morning walk and sun bath; weather and season permitting, morning meditation, connecting with God, your Creator, your Angels, the Masters etc.

- Drink at least 600mls water during this time.

- 1 White or green tea if desired.

Breakfast (approximately 8am)

- 1 apple or pear or 200 grams papaya or pineapple. (Breakfast on transitioning days will be very small)

Nothing for one hour after breakfast

Mid morning (approximately 10am)

- Add 1–2 tsp of green barley in organic grape juice, or fresh juice with 1/3 water. Drink small amounts of water throughout the morning totalling 1 litre before lunchtime.

Lunch

- 1 glass of water with the juice of half a lemon and 2 tsp vitamin C powder, 2 tsp liquid vitamins, eight drops of Cellfood, 2 capsules Co-Enzyme Q10, 1 Capsule Nutrition Diagnostics' Bio Zyme Formula.

20mins later:

- A large fruit salad (no melons) (See recipe section for suggestions). Top with almond cream (See recipe section).

- Go for a ten minute slow walk to help digestion; then rest a while.

Mid afternoon

- Add 1–2 tsp of green barley in organic grape juice, or fresh juice with 1/3 water. Drink small amounts of water throughout the morning totalling 1 litre before lunchtime.

- 1 white or green tea if desired.

Evening meal

- 1 glass of water with the juice of half a lemon and 2 tsp vitamin C powder.

- 1 Capsule Nutrition Diagnostics Bio Zyme Formula.

- 2 x Capsules EPA/DHA Omega 3

20mins later:

- A large vegetable salad with lots of organic large leafy greens, such as mixed lettuce, spinach, kale, or chard (See recipe section for suggestions). You can add a dressing of lemon juice, or rice vinegar with a little organic cold pressed olive oil mixed with a few herbs (See recipe section for suggestions).

NB: No dairy products allowed

During the transitioning days you can take in as many fresh juices and herbal teas as you like, as well as vegetable broth (See recipe section for suggestions). Make sure you allow time between drinking and eating for digestion. You must allow one to one and a half hours after eating and twenty minutes before eating.

Before Bed

- This is a good time to read spiritually inspired and uplifting books, do more meditation, and listen to relaxation music. Do not eat snacks. Give your body time to rest and rejuvenate, and to complete the elimination process. You do not want to waste energy digesting food or drink while you are sleeping.

It is important to go to bed early — no later than 9.30pm. Rest is imperative. If you are having trouble sleeping, particularly if you are used to going to bed late, this is a good time to meditate in bed and play relaxing music. Make sure the room is in total darkness; close curtains and blinds. If you still have trouble sleeping, ask your health care professional for a prescription for natural melatonin. This can be made up at a compound pharmacy or drug store.

Do Not: Take the melatonin straight off the shelf at the pharmacy or drug store, or health food store. In countries like Australia the amount of melatonin in the brands sold at pharmacies and health food stores is insufficient. Do not waste your money. Dosage requirements of Melatonin need to be verified by your health care practitioners.

If you have a daily sunbath; weather and season permitting, without sunglasses, the light will trigger the melatonin you need for a good night's sleep. Once you get used to not wearing sunglasses, your sleeping pattern will change thanks to the increased melatonin from sunlight. Sunbathing must be at times when it is safe. That is between sunrise and 10am, or after 3pm. At other times cover up, use organic 30plus sun block, and wear a hat and sunglasses with the exception of 10 to 15 minutes at midday especially for those living in area like United Kingdom.

* If using IntraMAX delete liquid vitamins, minerals and Cellfood. Take IntraMAX as per manufacturer's protocols.

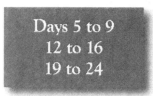

Days 5 to 9
12 to 16
19 to 24

Upon Rising

- Test your pH levels before taking any food or drink.

- Scrape your tongue and clean your teeth.

- This may also be a good time to do an enema, if you are not having colonics.

- Take Colozone as directed on the label followed by the juice of half a lemon in warm water and vitamin C.

Do not take Colozone on days when you have a colonic irrigation or on eating days.

30mins later

- Take Paracea, Probiotic and green barley in a little grape juice or water.

8am

- Fruit Juice diluted with one third filtered water. Add liquid vitamins, liquid minerals, 8 drops Cell Food.

10am

- Organic green tea or white tea.

12pm

- Vegetable juice diluted with one third filtered water. Add liquid vitamins, liquid minerals, 8 drops Cell Food.

2pm

- Organic green tea or white tea.

4pm

- Vegetable Juice diluted with filtered water. Add liquid vitamins, liquid minerals, 8 drops Cell Food.

6pm

- Broth. You can add a little Celtic salt and cayenne pepper to this.

8pm

- Juice of half a lemon and 2 tsp vitamin C in a small glass of water.

- This may also be a good time for your enema, if you are not having colonics.

Drink plenty of pure alkaline water throughout the day.

I provide juice and broth recipes in the recipe section at the end of this handbook.

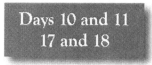

**Days 10 and 11
17 and 18**

Days 10 and 17

7am

- Juice of half a lemon and vitamin C, barley greens, Percy's Powder, Paracea, Probiotics.

8am

- Fruit juice diluted with one third filtered water. Add liquid vitamins, liquid minerals, 8 drops of Cell Food.

10am

- Organic green tea or white tea.

12 Midday

- One Capsule Bio-Zyme Formula to aid digestion together with the juice of half a lemon in one large glass of water.

12.30pm Lunch

You may eat a small raw salad at lunch time on days ten and eighteen; however, it must be completely raw as in the recipe below.

Suggested Ingredients:

60 grams mixed lettuce broken into small pieces together with a handful of baby spinach, 1 small carrot grated, 1 small beetroot grated, 1 roma tomato or 4 cherry tomatoes chopped in small portions, red onion finely chopped, handful of basil, mint, and parsley finely chopped, handful mung beans, handful sunflower seed sprouts, handful broccoli sprouts, 1 finely chopped stick of celery, half avocado, 4 sun dried organic tomatoes. Toss these ingredients in a bowl together with a dressing of your choice (no dairy). There are dressing recipes in the recipe section. Eat your food slowly and chew each mouthful at least twenty to thirty times.

4pm

- Organic green tea or white tea.

6pm

- Broth. You can add a little Celtic salt and cayenne pepper.

8pm

- Juice of half a lemon together with 1 tsp vitamin C in a small glass of water.

Days 11 and 18

7am

- Add to a glass of water the juice of half a lemon, and vitamin C, barley greens, Percy's Powder, Paracea, Probiotics and 2 Tbls of coconut oil.

8am

- 1 capsule Bio-Zyme Formula to aid digestion.

8.30am Breakfast

- Start with fruit — papaya, pineapple, kiwifruit and some berries, at least three colour varieties. Do not use any berries unless they are either organic or chemical free.

- Top your fruit with 2 Tbls S.L.A.P.S.B. (sunflower seeds, linseeds, almonds, pepitas, sesame seeds and Brazil nuts - see recipe section). These seeds and nuts should be ground. But if you do not have a suitable grinder; then soak them overnight in filtered water.

- 1 tsp Bee pollen.

- 2 Tbls organic desiccated coconut or organic coconut oil. This is optional. Do not add coconut oil if you have already added it to your morning lemon juice.

- 1 dsp Living Valley Springs Breakfast Herbs. You may find these herbs bitter to begin with, so start with one tsp and gradually increase the amount.

- 1 tsp Organic Maca.

- 1 handful organic raw oats (optional).

- Grated ginger (optional).

Top with organic coconut milk or organic yoghurt or organic non dairy milk.

Also

- 1 or 2 organic poached eggs. You may add a little Celtic salt and cayenne pepper, but not black or white pepper.

- Grilled tomato, avocado drizzled with balsamic dressing (see recipes).

- Serve with organic sour dough bread or waffles (see recipes).

  If you are on a candida regime replace fruit with a fresh salad comprising:Mixed lettuce, rocket, spinach, tomatoes, cucumber, grated carrot, avocado, onion, asparagus with dressing.

11am
- Organic green tea or white tea.

12.00pm
- 1 Capsule Bio-Zyme Formula to aid digestion together with the juice of half a lemon in one glass of water.

12.30pm
- A fresh salad. See recipe section in this book for suggestions.

This meal should be taken with vegetarian protein such as chickpea patties, walnut burgers, or potato and lentil pie. See recipe section under Mains or get more recipes in 'From Cancer to Wellness Cookbook'.

4pm
- Organic green tea or white tea.

6pm
- Broth. You may add a little Celtic salt and Cayenne pepper.

8pm
- Add to one glass of water the juice of half a lemon with 1 tsp vitamin C.

Days 25 to 28

Follow the same regime as on days one to four with the exception of the following:

- Stop enemas and colonics.

- In order to stimulate peristaltic activity (action of the bowel), take two Living Valley Springs Life Capsules on day 25 before breakfast. They contain aloe vera, myrrh and ginger.

OR

On days twenty five to twenty eight add to a cup of warm water, 1 tbls of bran such as oat, rice, or wheat. To this add 1 tbls of linseeds that have been soaked overnight. Linseeds; also known as flaxseed has a healing effect on the lining of the stomach and intestines as well as reinitiates peristaltic activity.

- Make sure you drink at least 2 litres of water EVERY DAY.

- The times for meditation, reading, journal writing, colonics, and enemas are only suggestions and can be adjusted to suit your lifestyle.

- The times for ColoZone, juicing and taking of any food or beverages should be adhered to.

- If you are working you must take time off to complete this cleanse. You cannot be committed to this program if you continue to put yourself in stressful circumstances and polluted environments while your body is detoxing.

- There are recipes at the back of the book for broths, juices, fruit salads, nut creams, vegetable salads, and dressings.

- Use good quality protein particularly organic eggs to increase the elimination of toxins.

- Lightly steam crucifer vegetables to release their anti-cancer properties.

- Tomatoes can also be cooked. Cooking releases Lycopene, a powerful antioxidant.

- Do not juice papaya, bananas, and strawberries as they do not dilute or liquefy enough.

- When juicing add one third the volume of filtered water to the juice.

- If you have access to a steam sauna or an infrared sauna, treat yourself whenever possible. This helps remove toxins from the body through the skin. Rub yourself gently with a long-haired, vegetable-fibre bristle brush to remove dead skin and toxins. This also stimulates the blood flow and assists the body's circulatory system. You can get these brushes from health food stores. Remember to have a cool shower after a sauna to close the pores of the skin.

Why juice?

Juicing allows your body to rest and work on the beneficial effects of the nutrients you are now giving your body to heal. Juicing also removes the indigestible fibre, making these nutrients more readily available to the body in much larger quantities than when eating a piece of fruit or a vegetable, because many nutrients are trapped in the fibre. This is one reason to purchase a slow juicer, so these nutrients are not destroyed by friction. Juicing is extremely beneficial, for example, the human body only assimilates 1% of the nutrient 'beta carotene' from a carrot when eaten whole, in comparison to 100% when the carrot is juiced'. (ref: www.living-foods.com)

Juicing assists with detoxifying the body. It also alleviates allergies, aids digestion, relieves high blood pressure, and contributes to a longer life expectancy. Keeping the body alkaline with juicing is known to reduce stress. Juicing strengthens the immune system to prevent and heal disease. It is one of the best tools that work immediately on the body. Everyone needs to juice yearly for a period of no less than 4 days and usually best for a period of 10 days. This gives the body a time out in order to rejuvenate.

Why should you eat in the middle of a juice fast?

The answer is that proteins and raw food taken in the middle of a fast help the liver to dump toxins.

To get the most out of this program you will need to invest not only your energy and time but also a little money.

This is a **true investment** for life. I can assure you that you will need all the tools recommended. They will not be hidden away in the cupboard after you complete the first 28 days of this program. You will use them for many years and so will your family and friends.

Equipment needed for Good Health Practices:

One Juicer: Many different juicers are on the market, but they are not all the same. Some are more efficient than others; I prefer the '**Compact Multi Purpose Juicer and Mincer' or 'Omega'**

These juicer are very versatile, and most affordable. They will juice wheat grass and make yummy fruit ice cream, as well as puree food and make nut butters, pasta, and noodles. Both capabke as a sausage maker, and can be used for dressings, dips, salsa and vegie patties. Both juicers are 'cold press masticating juicers' that produces high quality, living juice and makes the maximum of nutrients available, unlike high speed juicers which produce an oxygenated juice, heated at the molecular level. This shortens the life and quality of the juice.

One Food Processor: I prefer the **'Vita Mix Total Nutrition Centre'.**

'Vita Mix' performs 35 food processes — 2 to 30 times faster than other appliances, without attachments. 'Vita-Mix' maximises nutritional intake: It makes wonderful 'smoothies', soups, ice cream and can be used as a grinder/mill for nuts and seeds.

and/or

One Bamix Swissline Delux Blender 240W: This machine has a wet/dry mill attachment for grinding nuts and seeds plus a 900ml jug. It is an alternative for the Vita Mix at a much lower price. Google "Bamix Swissline Delux Blender" for your nearest stockist.

One Tongue Scraper: You can purchase these from the pharmacy, drug store, internet provider or dentist.

First thing in the morning, before you even take a drink of water, scrape your tongue. During cleansing, toxins find their way to your tongue during the night, particularly the back of your tongue. Scraping off the white or yellow toxic build up deposited on the tongue is most important. Use an inverted spoon if you cannot find a tongue scraper and scrape as far back on the surface of the tongue as you can without gagging. Then clean your teeth. This will help reduce bad breath, and the reintroduction of accumulated bacteria and toxins into your system.

You may experience increased 'drooling' at night as the body removes toxins through saliva while you are sleeping. This may leave a bad smell on your pillow, so take precautions to protect your linen.

One large stainless steel pot: with the capacity of six litres or six quarts. <u>Avoid aluminum.</u>

This is used to make a potassium broth for daily consumption, together with juices.

A sexy long 8 to 10 oz glass: to drink your juice and feel special!

If you do not have a really great long glass for your juices, treat yourself! By using a special glass, you are more likely to sit and sip, instead of swilling it down in a rush. You should focus on what you are doing, and why.

I use this time to take my mind to a memory of a holiday or to a great place and pretend I am drinking a cocktail. This works every time to change my day, and improve my well-being. Drink your juice or broth sitting in the sunshine early in the morning if possible for at least 20 minutes Or sit in the house where the sun is shining through an open window or door and enjoy your moment to heal yourself, while taking in the vitamin D and melatonin your body needs to heal.

Two dispensers of pH paper: These papers can be purchased from the United States. The coloured readings will show a pH from 4.5 to 8.5. You can register with their website as a regular customer and get the pH papers at a discounted price.

1. Go to www.microessentiallab.com.
2. Click on – Hydrion Saliva Urine pH test kits – Go to Catt# 2210 or Catt#345 and follow the prompts.

   For more information email custserv@microessentiallab.com.

One Journal: This is a great way to record your progress and to write your thoughts and affirmations; not to mention lots of little tips you will pick up on the way. Keep a file of all the information you collect as it may be helpful in the future, or for someone else. You will more than likely collect a vast amount of information about cancer from the internet, books, and magazines and from well wishing friends.

One Container of ColoZone: ColoZone is a natural supplement made up of magnesium oxide and magnesium carbonate. It releases oxygen into the digestive tract for cleansing and detoxification. ColoZone is manufactured from organic minerals which have been developed by NASA to obtain the maximum oxygen release (Molecular Cracking). ColoZone is a natural product for cleansing the system and supports colonics and enemas. Use while on the twenty eight day detox program.

ColoZone is to be taken on an empty stomach one and a half hours before consuming any food or drink. [On the container of the ColoZone the amounts to be taken are given for different body weights]

- Prepare the juice of half a lemon with 1000mg vitamin C in warm (not hot) water. Drink this immediately after ColoZone.

- Add 1 heaped teaspoon or more (depending on body weight) to half a glass of water. Stir thoroughly and drink followed by lemon juice and vitamin C.

- Repeat this every morning on juicing days according to 28 day program with the exception of days you choose to have a colonic or on days of consuming food. ColoZone can be purchased online or health food stores.

One Combination Douche/Enema with Water Bottle System: This can be bought at a drug store. You will need to use this one to two times a day while you are doing the juicing phase of this program if you are not having colonic irrigations. Go to www.thaiorganiclife.com to buy online.

Colonic Irrigation

If you have not had the 'pleasure' of a colonic irrigation previously, you are in for a wonderful experience as if you have had a shower on the inside. Colonic Irrigations will relieve some of the healing crisis symptoms some people experience; such as headaches and nausea. The benefits of knowing a 'good', caring professional to do this for you is invaluable.

If you are uncomfortable or unsure about using enemas by yourself, and would like a little pampering along the way, find a recommended Colonic Irrigation Practitioner. You will require a minimum of six Colonics — preferably ten Colonics (or more if you wish) during the juicing phase, particularly if you have not had a colon cleanse before.

During the juicing phase of your program; it is necessary to cleanse the bowel efficiently. This process alone may save your life. Removing harmful, breeding germs, bacteria and parasites is imperative if you plan to get well.

If you choose to go to a Colon Care Centre specialising in Colonic Irrigation, this is what you need to expect for your money: A good, qualified colon hydro-therapist will:

1. Allow at least one hour for the treatment.

2. Use filtered water at varying temperatures.

3. Gently massage your abdominals during each session.

4. Use approx. 25 litres of filtered water.

5. Carefully and considerately filter this water into your colon through a specifically designed apparatus which is sterilised and uses individually sealed packs of tubing, attached to a sterile, disposable speculum.

6. Introduce this water intermittently, in small amounts over this period of time, all the while, consulting you as to the comfort of the process and explaining what is happening and the benefits of the cleanse.

7. Introduce Lactobacilli back into the bowel at the end of each colonic.

This process will be slowly and carefully hydrating the bowel, whilst loosening faecal plaque and impacted faecal waste matter, thereby aiding elimination of toxins (including liver toxicity) gas blockages, undigested food and mucus.

No one involved has to smell or touch faecal matter with closed colonic irrigation, making the procedure extremely focused on safety, hygiene and comfort for the client and the practitioner. You will also be covered with a sheet or towel during the procedure.

For additional healing, coffee or herbs may be introduced for clients wanting greater cleansing. Your Practitioner will explain the benefits of each additive to your cleanse.

You will be lying on your side for insertion and on your back during most of the procedure, except when lactobacilli and herbs are added. You may need to go on to your side to hold these ingredients for a few minutes while they take effect.

The benefits of cleansing the colon include the following:

- Ridding the body of accumulated metabolic wastes and chemical toxins, thereby assisting the immune system to function optimally.

- Relief of headaches, lack of concentration, foggy head during the detox phase.

- Relief of liver overload and nausea.

- Relief from backache resulting from an overloaded colon.

- Relief from depression caused by toxins lingering in the system.

- Relief of irritable bowel syndrome, candida and yeast infections.

- Relief from constipation, bloating and flatulence as excess air and waste are removed.

- Supporting the elimination of parasites by eliminating the environment in which they breed.

- Relief with digestives problems as the system is cleaned and cleared.

- Relief of fatigue as the system can now function without wasted energy.

More information about colonic cleansing and care is available at: www. coloncarecentre.com.au/colonic.

If you choose not to do either an enema or colonic; your body will want to eliminate massive amounts of toxins/waste by re-absorption through the colon wall, adding toxins to the rest of your body through other avenues, such as the skin and urine. This can lead to nausea, headaches, fatigue and irritability and slow down and may even prevent the healing process.

Your commitment to cleaning out your body so it can absorb nutrition is most important. You will feel so much better afterward that you will wonder why you didn't do this type of cleanse on a regular basis all your life.

Skin Brushing

Dr Bernard Jensen DC, ND, who published over forty books in his sixty years as a pioneer in holistic health and healing states that skin brushing eliminates uric acid crystals and other various acids in the body. Our bodies make skin every twenty four hours. Dr Jensen believes the skin must be as clean as the blood is. Skin brushing removes the top layer of old skin, in turn removing waste acids. Use only a dry vegetable bristle brush. NEVER USE NYLON. Use the brush dry on the skin gently first thing in the morning before you shower or bath. You can purchase these brushes at most health food stores and some pharmacies or drug stores.

Nutritional Supplements:

The list of nutritional supplements on the following pages are suggested for everyone with any type of cancer. These products will either be in liquid or powder form, so that your digestive system can take a holiday for a few days, and your body can concentrate on healing when you are juicing. Digestion takes energy, liquid vitamins and minerals are absorbed easily into your system. This allows for faster regeneration.

Nutritional Supplements

SUPPLEMENT	DOSAGE	COMMENTS
Nature's Way Alive! Organic Vitamin C **or** **Nutrition Diagnostics Bio-Vitamin C**	2 tsp 3 times daily.	Gentle to the stomach, Naturally buffered, Easily Absorbed 100% Whole Food Complex, made from Fruit, USDA Organic Certified, Vegan. Made from four of Mother Nature's most potent organic fruit sources: Organic Acerola, Organic Goji, Organic Amla, Organic Kiwi. Ascorbic Acid, Lysine, Glycine, Proline, Citrus Bioflavonoids extract, green tea.
Probiotics **Nutrition Care Lactobac Powder** or similar	1 level tsp 2 times daily in juice or water.	Helps to maintain healthy digestive function and balances out the friendly bacteria of the stomach. **Active Ingredients:** Dairy free, *Lactobacillus rhamanosus* and *Bifidobacteria* Powder containing no less than 5 billion organisms per gram.
Percy's Powder Can be purchased from health food stores and some health care professionals	1 tsp daily with lemon juice and vitamin C powder.	Helps with alkalinity. **Active Ingredients:** Magnesium 78.1mg, Potassium 131mg, Iron (9.1mg, Zinc, 10.2mg, Manganese 9.1mg.
Good Liquid Multi Vitamin together with a Colloidal Mineral Preferably organic. See IntraMAX.	2 tsp three times daily in juice.	Active ingredients must be sugar and preservative free.

SUPPLEMENT	DOSAGE	COMMENTS
Bioceuticals Paracea Forte (If taking Paracea when juicing; break open capsules and dissolve in your daily lemon juice). or **Liquid Herbal Formula of Wormwood, Black Walnut together with cloves** — Most Health Food Stores carries this mixture or purchase from an Herbalist or Naturopath.	2 Capsules 3 times daily before meals, (breakfast, lunch and dinner).	Helps to maintain digestive function, and rid the body of parasites, worms, bacteria, and candida and gut disturbances. **Active Ingredients:** Artemisia Herb (Chinese Wormwood), Berberis vulgaris (Barberry), Stem bark, Juglans nigra (Black Walnut), Citrus x paradise (Grapefruit) fruit.
Organic Barley Greens	2 tsp or more into juice twice daily. Start with ½ tsp each day, gradually increasing to two or more teaspoons over a two week period — this will minimise any detoxification symptoms you may experience. (It is OK to take up to 12 or more teaspoons a day, which some people do. Sprinkle on cereal, mix with juice or water).	Barley Grass is a super food. It is alkalising to the body and helps with energy levels. **Alkalising Nutritional Information** Calcium, Magnesium Potassium, Sodium, Iron, Zinc, Acid Minerals, Sulphur, Phosphorus, Chlorine, A superoxide dismutase, a powerful antioxidant **Amino Acids:** Alanine, Amide, Arginine, Aspartic acid, Cystine, Glutamic Acid, Glycine, Histidine, Isoleucine, Leucine, Lysine, methionine, phenylalanine, Proline, Purines, Serine, Threonine, Tryptophan, Tyrosine, Valine, fatty acids and enzymes.
Organic Virgin Coconut Oil	3 Tbls once daily.	Organic Coconut Oil has an anti-carcinogenic effect on the body, and helps rid the body of tumors.

SUPPLEMENT	DOSAGE	COMMENTS
BioCeuticals Ultra Clean EPA/DHA plus or **Udo's Choice Certified Organic DHA Oil Blend*** or **Deva Organic Vegan Omega 3 with DHA*** *suitable for vegetarians.*	2 Capsules twice daily.	**Active Ingredients:** Concentrated Omega-3 Triglycerides-fish 994.6mg equiv. Eicosapentaenoic acid (EPA), 300mg Equiv. Docosahexaenoic acid (DHA) 200mg, D-alpha-Tocopherol 16.8mg (equiv. Natural Vitamin E 25IU)
Nutrition Diagnostics Bio-Zyme Formula or similar.	1 Capsule in between meals.	Promotes Digestion. See chart in Eradication Program for active ingredients.
Drs Best Co-Enzyme Q10 200mg or similar	3 Capsules x three daily (up to fifteen capsules can be taken).	Improves tissue oxygenation, supports immune system.

In the previous chart I have not added a brand name to the liquid vitamins and colloidal minerals. However, Hy-Vita Liquid Vitamin together with Bio Activ Volcomin is a good choice or Twintab's Vita Quick together with Mini Quick Liquid Minerals. Add Cellfood to this. Cellfood assists in the detoxification and oxygenates the body. Eight drops of Cellfood is taken three times a day in water or juice. My personal choice is the following 100 % carbon-bond organic product that can be used instead of the liquid vitamin, minerals, and Cellfood. I use these liquid vitamins and mineral combinations. It would be the best I have come across. Produced in the United States by Drucker Labs and developed by a Dr Richard Drucker.

IntraMAX

This is one product that covers all essential vitamins, minerals, oxygenates the body and assists in detoxification. This product is called IntraMAX. It is an organic all in one vitamin, mineral, complete food. It is important to use the manufacturer's protocols when taking this product due to its ability to detoxify the body. To buy IntraMAX go to the IntraMAX product page on www.Cleansurroundings.com. The product page also has many links to helpful information about IntraMAX, including protocols and ingredients. All Health Care Professionals can go direct to Drucker Labs. To Register go to www.druckerlabs.com or http://store.druckerlabs.com/v/HCPRegistration.aspx.

Intravenous (IV) Vitamin C

Together with the list of nutritional supplements listed, I would like to suggest that you have regular Intravenous (IV's) vitamin C infusions. Vitamin C IV's supplies over 1000 (micromol/litre) and reaches the blood stream 25% faster than taking vitamin C by mouth.

It has been reported that higher doses such as these do not work as an antioxidant; they work as an oxidizer and scavenger and kills off cancer cells and viruses. Vitamin C infusions have been described as a "Smart Bomb" by medical practitioners using this method.

How to get Vitamin C Intravenous Injections?

A doctor or a hospital in most countries will give these infusions if you ask. Most medical practitioners working in the field of anti-ageing, holistic, integrative and nutritional medicine will have a supply of vitamin C IV's on hand, or they will order the amount required.

Suggested Protocols

Four IV's of 60–100 grams in the first week followed by five IV's of 50 grams the following week. I recommend more rather than less. You can also take another five 50 gram IV's over 2 days if you wish. Confirm the amount with your health care professional who may have a different opinion. My research and experience supports higher rather than lower doses of vitamin C IV's. You cannot overdose on vitamin C.

I can assure you vitamin C IV's work, not only on cancer but also on many other chronic conditions such as cardiovascular disease, asthma, herpes zoster (shingles), candida, diabetes mellitus type I and II, HIV, multiple sclerosis, rheumatoid arthritis, chronic fatigue syndrome and related viruses, migraine headaches, bacterial infections and the list goes on.

Some patients who go for the Splash Poison Burn therapy are told to avoid vitamin C as it will interfere with the poison their misguided doctors are going to give them. Remove the poison and patients will have a much better rate of survival and are more likely to live a long healthy life especially if they implement the nutritional guidelines in this book.

It has been alleged that vitamin C creates kidney stones and strips B12 from the body. This is untrue, but unfortunately there are still many practitioners who will try to convince you of this. These accusations have been proven to be false.

Once you have completed the twenty eight days you will be ready for the Optimum Daily Program. This is a program I have set out for you in order to maintain health. It provides suggested menus and nutritional supplementation. Some of the supplements can be decreased over a period of three to six months. See tumor marker tests.

Notes

RECOMMENDED OPTIMUM DAILY PROGRAM

On rising	Test pH Levels: this must be done prior to any food or liquid. 1 large glass of warm water with the juice of half a lemon. **To this add:** 2 tsp of liquid vitamins, 2 tbls minerals, or IntraMAX according to protocols. 2 tsp powdered vitamin C. 1 heaped tsp probiotic. 2 tbls organic coconut oil. 1 sachet of Percy's Powder. 1 heaped tsp Barley Greens. 2 capsules EPA/DHA 2 glasses of water up to 30 mins before breakfast.
Breakfast **Suggestion # 1**	Fresh fruit at least 3 varieties and colours 2 tbls SLAPSB (See recipe section). Avoid peanuts. 2 tbls desiccated coconut. 1 tsp organic bee pollen. 1 dsp Living Valley Springs Breakfast Herbs, 1 tsp maca powder, grated ginger, A handful raw oats (optional). Top with coconut milk or yoghurt. **Also:** Poached, scrambled or soft boiled eggs with grilled tomato and avocado with dressing (see recipes) or a plain omelet topped with Celtic salt and cayenne pepper. Do not use black or white pepper. Serve the eggs on one of the following grains: millet, buckwheat, brown rice, quinoa, or oats. Alternatively use spelt flours or sour dough breads.

Breakfast Suggestion #2	Poached, scrambled, or soft boiled eggs or an Omelet with mushrooms, onion, garlic, tomato, asparagus, and parsley **To this add:** Fresh salad vegetables including mixed lettuce, rocket, spinach, tomatoes, cucumber, grated carrot, avocado, olives, feta or vegan cheese, olives and salad dressing. Optional add: Steamed vegetables, broccoli, brussels sprouts, carrots, topped with cold pressed olive oil.	
Breakfast Supplements	2 Capsules CO Enzyme Q10. 1ml Selenium. 1 Capsule Nutrition Diagnostics Bio-Zyme Formula.	
Mid Morning	No food or fluids for at least 1 ½ hours after breakfast. Then drink 1 litre of pure water before lunch. Drink this water in regular small amounts. 2 capsules Bioceuticals Quercetin, containing Quercetin/Bromelain or similar. 1 cup of green or white tea. Fresh juice diluted with 1/3 volume of water with 1 tsp barley greens.	**Test pH Levels prior to mid morning vitamins (2 hours after breakfast).**
30 Mins before Lunch	1 glass of water with juice of half a lemon. **Add:** 2 tsp powdered vitamin C.	
Lunch Suggestion	Protein foods. Choose from eggs, lentils, chickpea patties, humus, tempeh, miso, a variety of legumes. With: Fresh salad vegetables, sprouts, and dressing (see recipe section in this book) Soft cheeses. Choose from feta, camembert, brie, cottage, and ricotta. Celtic salt and cayenne pepper, if desired. Organic sour dough bread, cracker bread or wraps.	
Lunch Supplements	2 capsules CO Enzyme Q10. 1 Capsule Nutrition Diagnostics Bio-Zyme Formula.	

Mid Afternoon	No food or fluids for at least 1 ½ hours after lunch. Then drink 1 litre of pure water before dinner. Drink this water in regular small amounts. 2 capsules Bioceuticals Quercetin (containing Quercetin/Bromelain) or similar. 1 cup green or white tea.	

30 Mins before Dinner	1 Glass of water with juice of half lemon. **Add:**
	
	   2 tsp powdered vitamin C.
	
	   1 heaped teaspoon probiotic.
	
	   2 Capsules EPA/DHA	

Dinner
 	
Suggestions
	Choose one of the following:
	
	   1 cup miso soup.
	
	   Fresh vegetable juice.
	
	   Protein shake.
	
	   Potassium broth.
	
	   Vegetable sticks and humus.
	
	   Homemade soup.
	
	   Fresh salad.
	
	   Steamed vegetables.	

Dinner Supplements	1 capsules Nutrition Diagnostics Bio-Zyme Formula or similar.	
Before Bed	Melatonin or a natural sleep tonic if needed (take as prescribed). A warm soak in a bath with a few drops of clary sage or similar. This is a good time for meditation & reading of inspiring and uplifting books.	

Helpful Suggestions	<ul><li>Sprouts can be included in all salads wherever possible — especially broccoli.</li><li>Follow an exercise program that suits your general daily routine.</li><li>Meditate daily. You may like to join a meditation group or prayer group.</li><li>Go for an early morning walk and do stretch exercises.</li><li>Find a good, caring, personal trainer, preferably a trainer qualified in rehabilitation.</li><li>Laugh a lot, watch funny movies, and listen to uplifting music.</li><li>Avoid loud and aggressive people.</li><li>Avoid hostile situations and confrontations to reduce your stress level.</li><li>Surround yourself with loving, caring, gentle and spiritually aware people who are concerned about your wellbeing.</li><li>Be gentle with yourself.</li><li>Visualise the cells in your body as being healthy.</li><li>Have Faith.</li><li>Affirm your positivity; use affirmations.</li><li>Believe in yourself and be determined to succeed.</li></ul>	

ALL profits made from products manufactured and carrying the label of **Living Valley Springs (LVS)** are donated to benevolent work to relieve sickness and suffering in Australia and overseas, including orphanages in East Africa.

Go to www.lvs.com.au to buy their products online.

Additional information:

Maca is an excellent product. It improves stamina, strength and energy, and it is also a hormonal tonic. Add it to water, juice, cereals, smoothies, yoghurt or herbal teas. Take 1/2 to 2 teaspoons six days a week (have one day off). Like super foods, such as green barley, wheat grass and bee pollen, maca helps to alkaline the urine thereby helping to mobilise toxins in the body.

Fresh Organic Ginger is a powerful antioxidant. It cleanses the colon, and stimulates circulation. It also fights inflammation, and works as a blood thinner. Ginger contains phytochemicals, amino acids, essential fatty acids, cucumin, selenium, zinc, vitamins B1, B2, B3, B6, C and A. Ginger is an amazing plant. But it is best not to use ginger if you are taking anticoagulant drugs, or if you have gallstones. Good quality organic ginger is a replacement for aspirin used and recommended to patients by many general practitioners to thin the blood.

Breakfast Herbs

One of my favourite products from LVS is their **Breakfast Herbs.** These herbs are a little bitter to start with, but your taste buds get used to it. Start with a 1/4 teaspoon and build up to 1 dsp daily.

LVS Herbs contain the following seven herbs:
(This information comes from one of their handouts)

Astragalus: *Astragalus membranaceus* is a tonic for building both vitality and blood. It is antiviral because it increases immunity and the amount of interferon. Astragalus also increases the function of natural killer (NK) cells and counters the immunosuppressant effects of cortisone. A clinical study of one thousand people showed that Astragalus protects against the common cold.

Withania: *Withania somnifera* is a herb that is indigenous to India. It is used as a general tonic, and in the treatment of nervous disorders. Withania is an adaptogenic herb. An adaptogen is a substance that has a non-specific action in increasing resistance to various stresses including physical, chemical and biological. It is relatively innocuous and normalises biological functions.

Slippery Elm: Protects against irritations and inflammations of the mucous membranes. It is used whenever people have difficulty holding and digesting food. Slippery elm contains vitamins E, F, K, and P as well as iron, sodium, calcium, selenium, iodine, copper, zinc and some potassium and phosphorus.

Bacopa: Bacopa is a traditional Ayurvedic herb. It is used as a brain tonic to improve memory and learning abilities. It promotes longevity, and fights nervous deficit from injury or stroke. Other traditional uses include the treatment of epilepsy, nervous breakdown and exhaustion.

St Mary's Thistle: *Silybum marianum* has been used traditionally for chronic liver disease. More recently it has been found to be effective wherever any chemical or drug abuse threatens normal liver function. St Mary's Thistle is one of the few herbs capable of regenerating liver cells.

Siberian Ginseng: Contains essential vitamins, mineral salts and amino acids. Consequently, it is of great value to the human organism. The plant is used principally to combat viral and bacterial infection. It does this by enhancing immune action. It has a tonic effect on cardiovascular function, improving athletic performance and energy output. Siberian Ginseng helps to normalise blood sugar levels.

Licorice Root: Licorice Root is one of the most versatile herbs with many therapeutic properties that work in synergy with other herbs to increase their effectiveness. Some of its benefits lie in its unique anti-viral properties, anti-inflammatory action and its tonic effect on the adrenal glands.

Optional Additional Nutritional Supplements

The additional optional nutritional supplements on the following page may be needed in your daily intake according to the type of cancer. A definition of terms used follow on the next page.

TYPE OF CANCER	NUTRIENT
Basal cell carcinoma	Selenium
Bladder	Activated B6 selenium, genistein
Brain	Vitamins, D3, CLA, GLA, K2, K3, GLA, CLA, selenium.
Breast	Activated B6, Indole-3-Carbinol, CLA, selenium, Pyridoxal-5-phosphate, D-glucaric acid, genistein.
Cervical	Indole-3-Carbinol, Activated B6, Resveratrol, Pyridoxal-5-phosphate, selenium.
Colon	Selenium, Modified Citrus Pectin, Choline, D-glucaric acid, D3, A, CLA, genistein.
Endometrial	B6, selenium.
Leukemia	Vitamins A, K, D3, Activated B6, E, Resveratrol, genistein, selenium.
Liver	Choline, selenium, GLA, cucumin.
Lung	Selenium, Activated B6, A, D3.
Lymphoma	Vitamin A, selenium.
Melanoma	Activated B6, A, D3, genistein, selenium, CLA, Resveratrol, melatonin, Modified Citrus Pectin.
Oesophageal	Selenium, genistein.
Oral	Selenium.
Osteosarcoma	Vitamin A, D3 and selenium.
Ovarian	Vitamin A, selenium, genistein, folic acid.
Pancreatic	Selenium, Resveratrol, Pyridoxal-5-phosphate.
Prostate	Vitamin D3, Zinc, selenium, Indole-3-Carbinol, Modified Citrus Pectin, CLA, genistein.
Skin	Vitamin B3, GLA, selenium.
Stomach	Genistein, selenium, Modified Citrus Pectin.
Uterine	Vitamin A, selenium, folic acid.
All cancers	Mitochondrial nutrients such as Co Enzyme Q10 are most important, together with Lipoic Acid and selenium, GLA/EFA, niacin, vitamin E (Tocopheryl succinate form) all help to normalise cancer cells.

Folic acid repairs DNA mutation in most cancers. |

Definitions

CLA: Conjugated linoleic acid is a powerful anticarcinogen and is reported to reduce metastasis.

GLA: Gamma linolenic acid is an omega 6 fatty acid and used to reduce metastasis.

Indol-3-Carbinol: An antioxidant that can stimulate natural detoxifying enzymes in the body. It occurs naturally in cruciferous vegetables like broccoli, cabbage, kale, and so on. Indol-3-Carbinol protects against breast and cervical cancer thanks to the way it breaks down estrogen.

Resveratrol: A powerful antioxidant found in the skin and seeds of grapes, blueberries, and other fruits. It helps to prevent cell damage and to normalise cancer cells.

Pyridoxal-5-phosphate: Inhibits the formation of tumors, and breaks down fats, protein and carbohydrates in food.

Modified Citrus Pectin: Helps prevent cancer metastasis, improves bowel flora, acts as a dietary fibre, and stimulates the immune system.

D-Glucaric Acid: An important nutrient found in fruit and vegetables. D-Glucaric Acid eliminates harmful toxins and reduces circulating levels of estrogen.

Choline: Protects the liver from all types of cellular damage, and can reverse damage that has already occurred.

Folic Acid: Repairs DNA mutation in most cancers.

Genistein: A strong antioxidant that removes damaging free radicals and reduces lipid peroxidation. Genistein has been known to reduce the risk of some hormone-related cancers, principally breast and prostate cancer. Genistein seems also to inhibit the activity of tyrosine kinase, which plays a role in cell growth. If Tyrosine is reduced so is the risk of cancer. It has anti-estrogen action. Genistein binds with estrogen receptors, preventing and inhibiting cancer growth.

Cucumin (Turmeric): An antioxidant able to prevent free radicals forming and to neutralize existing free radicals. It has the ability to stop cells from changing within the DNA; it also interferes with the enzymes necessary for cancer to progress. Cucumin is a pefect substitute for pain relief for those needing this kind of support. Cucumin should not be taken by those taking anticoagulants.

You may ask why you need to take supplements at all if your new diet is healthy and your life style has changed for the better. The answer is simple. If you have cancer, your body is depleted of nutrients. For a while at least, you need to boost your delicate system so that your body can heal. If you live in a polluted environment, which most of us do, nutritional supplements are essential. You can however discontinue many of the supplements after about three to six months. Have a tumor marker blood test, also called a cancer marker test first and an **MRI** (Magnetic Resonance Imaging) to make sure you are clear.

What is a Cancer (Tumor) Marker Test?

'*Tumor markers are substances, usually protein, that are produced by the body in response to cancer growth, or by the tissue itself. Some Tumor markers are specific for one type of cancer, while others are seen in several cancer types'* (Lab Tests Online UK — a public resource on clinical lab testing from the laboratory professionals who do the testing). The following is a list of Marker tests carried out by pathologists:

Breast:	CA 15.3, CEA
Colon:	CA 19.9, CEA
Liver:	AFP (Alpha fetoprotein)
Lung:	CEA, Mesomark
Myeloma, CCL:	Beta 2 Microglobulin
Ovary:	CA 125
Cervical:	CA 125
Prostate:	Free PSA, PSA
Stomach:	CA, 19.9, CEA
Pancreas:	CA, 19.9, CEA
Bile Ducts:	CA, 19.9, CEA
Testicular:	AFP, Beta HCG

There is also the Darkfield Microscopy that allows doctors to view blood cells to see how healthy the cells are. Many Naturopaths and alternative physicians often use this approach to check on an individual's condition.

DR-70 blood test can screen for 13 different types of cancers at the same time. Cancers that can be detected by this method are Breast, Cervix, Colon, Esophagus, Liver, Lung, Malignant Lymphoma, Ovary, Pancreas, Rectum, and Thyroid Cancer.

When all is clear keep up the Optimum Recommended Daily Program. This will become second nature to you as your taste buds will change and the thought of eating rubbish will not by now enter your consciousness. This program, will not only be part of you being cancer free, it will also be part of a maintenance lifestyle where healthy choices will keep you fit and disease free.

I have provided many recipes for you to use and to get you started.

The Lifestyle Guidelines section which follows is about the art of mind power. There are tips on getting benefit from exercise, the sun, and how to choose a good personal trainer.

LIFESTYLE GUIDELINES

'What we are today comes from our thoughts of yesterday,
and our present thoughts build our life of tomorrow:
*Our life is the creation of our mind' – **the Buddha***

We have been gifted with the ability to take charge of our thoughts, and our thought processes. Each day can be a wonderful experience when we choose to use our mind more effectively. We all have the ability to change what we do and the way we react to all situations that come into our life. We are the masters of our future. We can by using the power of intention program our mind and body to heal. You need to formulate what you want and not be influenced by all that exists around you.

Taking back your power

From the time we are born we give our power to others. As a baby, we do not have a choice. Unfortunately most of us stay controlled by our surroundings, upbringing and relationships. We often allow others to make the decisions for us. Doctors are notorious for putting pressure on their patients to take drugs which work on the effects of diseases instead of treating the causes. An oncologist told me to 'get my affairs in order' because I was going to die in less than 12 months. If I had accepted his opinion then that is what would have happened. I would be dead! Instead I took control and cured myself by going back to nature and changing my thoughts and my reactions. I was determined not to listen to those who where negative or encouraging me to be fearful. Placing myself in a bubble of protection I stood strong against all odds.

Attitudes of the medical industry

Many of you will suffer ridicule from some of the representatives of the medical industry, as I did, if you refuse to participate in the Splash, Poison and Burn (SPB) type of treatment. Stand in your own power and use your mind to overcome the negativity and fear these doctors may place upon you. They may mean well, but unfortunately their training does not recognise natural nutrition or exercising the God-given power of the mind.

Remember too that doctors do not have the right to tell you that you are going to die. Nor may they employ fear tactics to influence you to accept SPB treatment. Aboriginals used to point the bone at their enemies. This is a form of black magic intended to project fear, illness and death. A victim who believed the curse suffered restlessness, agitation, sleeplessness, trauma and very often death. If you have been told to get your affairs in order and the only treatment for you is SPB, then you will need to use your mind to overcome these negative *pointing the bone* suggestions.

Acid stress

Healing does not only depend on nutrition. We must also learn to manage our stress levels by taking back our power. After all, stress and anxiety comes from a belief that something bad is about to happen in our lives. Our bodies become acidic when we are unable to control our stress. Our emotions are linked to our immune system. If we want to strengthen our immune system then we need to eliminate negative elements in our life and thought processes.

Being grateful and giving thanks

Be grateful for all the gifts bestowed upon you, even the gift of cancer. This is an awakening and a time to walk a path different from the one you have been on. Your commitment to faith, hope, courage and love, together with your determination will be a guiding light for others to follow. Your family and friends will benefit from you showing them the way.

Smile and the whole world will smile with you

Keep a smile on your face and in your heart. This is a foundation for healing on its own. Anger, intolerance, and fear lead to disease and an early death.

The power of affirmations

Affirmations are a wonderful way of controlling the subconscious mind. Affirmations are positive statements that change the way you think about yourself and your health.

Since the unconscious mind cannot tell the difference between a real or imagined idea, it responds to whatever suggestions you give it, eventually helping to create the reality that matches your most predominant beliefs, attitudes, and thoughts. By repeating positive affirmations you can retrain your mind to feel more confident, as well as improve your overall health. (www.theholisticshop.com)

It is important when saying or writing affirmations that you relate them to the NOW. For instance: 'I am **NOW** healthy and free of pain and disease' or 'I **NOW** feel healthy and full of vigour'. By placing the word **NOW** in every affirmation you are placing your needs and desires in the **NOW**, not in the future.

> **'Today, I NOW view every experience as a blessing**
>
> **and a remedy that serves my well being,**
>
> **my healing path now exists within me,**
>
> **I love, trust and approve of myself'**

(Adapted from a Caroline Myss quotation to form a positive affirmation)

Speak affirmations out loud, and write them down ten times or more in a journal. I have kept a journal since I was diagnosed with cancer. I am most grateful for being led to this type of expression. Without it this book might not have been written.

Remember too; speak to yourself and others with love and watch your thoughts. If you find yourself thinking negatively or in a stressful situation, that is a good time to write down a positive affirmation. If you are not in a position to write one down, or to say it out loud, just think it. Place yourself in a bubble of white light to deflect negativity, and to regain positivity in your heart and mind.

We are confronted every day with attitudes and energies of others. You can be the light in the dark. Laughter and a happy genuine smile will negate all negative thoughts, and actions. The power of joy is a strong emotion. Be joyful and avoid imposing expectations onto others. That only produces hurt, pain and resentment.

The power of forgiveness

Louise Hay states that cancer is created through 'Deep hurt and longstanding resentment, deep secrets or grief eating away at the self. Carrying hatreds.'

Most of us can relate to this at some point in our life.

Nurturing me back to health required me not only to take care of my nutrition but also to correct my 'emotional nutrition'. Forgiveness and dealing with grief are the first steps to health and wellbeing. Here is a way to achieve this.

Write down a list of all the people that have hurt you, not forgetting yourself. Include unresolved grief and unhappy events.

Light a candle

Sit or lie in a comfortable position, light a candle and close your eyes. Take in a deep breath, expanding your diaphragm, and hold it for the count of 3. Let the air out slowly for the count of 5. Make sure your body is relaxed. Put on relaxing music if you wish and leave it playing softly in the background.

Visualise either a person or event that has caused you hurt. Create a ball of light in your hands and send this ball of light together with love to the heart of the person or event that has hurt you. Say and visualise the following:

'I NOW send the power of love, light and forgiveness within my heart to the heart of (speak or write in the person's name or the event) and I send it forth on a violet flame'.

Now you can visualise this violet flame reaching the heart of the person or the situation. Watch it expand to cover the person or event in question, and then bring back the love and light to yourself. Forgive yourself in the same way.

The exercise above can be done as often as you like. In addition use the affirmation 'I NOW lovingly forgive (name of person or event)'. This is very helpful in this situation and truly works. I suggest that you also write these actions in your journal. This will enable you to look back and see just how far you have come from the days when you were stuck in the past.

These exercises will feel foreign to many of you. But just go with it and trust in the power of the spoken word and the thoughts we carry around with us. They can either heal or destroy you.

Trust in the power of your creator and the angels

Involving yourself in spiritual work by going to church, making a sanctuary within your home, or out in nature can be extremely healing for your soul and beneficial for your physical and emotional wellbeing.

In 1985 my husband Wayne was instrumental in my discovery of the benefits of correct nutrition. He had cured himself of cancer four years before we met. He did this through nutrition, mental imaging, meditation and visualisation techniques, and the belief in God, Angels, Nature Spirits, and The Masters.

This same path has led me to be the person I am today: strong, determined, and always living with hope, faith and a feeling of abundance no matter what life throws at me. I sometimes stumble and falter, but I get back up, dust myself off, and start all over again. Faith helps rid yourself of fear, and gives you an immense power over everything that happens in your life. Faith has different meanings to many people. According to the Wikipedia Encyclopedia, *faith is a belief in the trustworthiness of an idea*. Used informally, the meaning can be quite broad, and may be used instead of either "trust", "belief" or "hope". As with trust, faith involves a concept of future events or outcomes.

Most importantly, you must have faith and belief in yourself. If this is lacking then work hard on overcoming barriers. These impede the natural flow of achievement. To me faith is an inner knowing. No matter what your upbringing or convictions, connecting with your creator is one of the most important steps toward the natural laws of health. Connecting with God, your Angels or connecting with nature and all that it provides, strengthens you to forgive and thus heal.

Receiving

Be open to receive. How many of you find it easy to give but when it comes to receiving, you block the flow? Some of you feel embarrassed when a kind act is done for you. Some of you feel guilty, as if you do not deserve help and attention. Believe me, if you are trying to heal yourself of cancer, this is not a time to feel too independent. Women are notorious for their inability to receive. They have been indoctrinated through the ages to be only givers and care takers. So do not hesitate to receive gifts – physical gifts, spiritual gifts, or gifts of money.

The power of hypnotherapy for relaxation

'Hypnotherapy is a technique that bypasses the conscious mind to the subconscious mind to help facilitate emotional or attitudinal change. Hypnotherapy is used to treat stress, phobias, and many other therapeutic needs to promote healing. Hypnotherapy is often used in counseling and by psychotherapists to help a client overcome psychological or physical problems'. (www.google.com.au/search?define:hypnotherapy).

It is a safe way of reaching your subconscious mind. Movies, television programs and comic books often portray hypnosis as evil and mind controlling. This is not true. Self hypnosis is valuable for highly stressed individuals.

I can highly recommend the relaxation CD's of Glenn Harrold. Glenn has a very pleasant English accent and guides you into a deeply relaxing state of mind and body. His CD's contain powerful subliminal suggestions that compound the overall effects. There is a CD in Glenn's collection that is on motivation and energy. This is helpful if you feel you are going off track.

The power of meditation, visualisation, and mental imaging

Meditation enables us to gain a clear perception of what we believe, and to release old patterns and beliefs we no longer need. Meditation is a journey of self-discovery which helps us relax and become free of stress and pain. Meditation uses the mind. It can align our chakras and so establish a direct channel to our Soul and to the source of all creation.

The word 'chakra' is derived from a Sanskrit word meaning 'wheel' and we are made up of seven major chakras starting at the base of the spine. The chakras connect with the body to our physical organs and systems as well as our emotions. For more information about the chakras google 'What are chakras'. There are plenty of sites dedicated to this. Also a beginners book which is helpful is 'Chakras for Beginners' written by David Pond.

Using mental imaging, we can focus our mind on the cells of our body, and see them in a state of perfection. Meditation does not necessarily have a spiritual or a religious aspect. It helps you take control of your body and mind.

How to meditate

The following is an easy method of meditation:

Find a place you can relax and not be disturbed. You can place some relaxing music on and light a candle. You may also like to light incense. I do both.

Sit up straight in a comfortable chair or lie down on a bed or the floor. You may like to go outdoors under a tree, in a park or on the beach. Whatever your choosing, it must be somewhere comfortable, try not to fall asleep though. Close your eyes. Shake out the stress, and relax your shoulders and body. Now concentrate on your breathing. This is extremely important. You must do diaphragmatic breathing. To do this, take a deep breath in through your nose, expanding your diaphragm, and hold for the count of 3, then slowly exhale through your mouth to the count of 5.

Breathing in through your nose and out through your mouth may take a little time to get used to. Repeat this until you can feel your body relax. Five times is usually enough. Breathing in this way allows your mind and body to become peaceful and aware and ready for visualisation.

Another method is to count steps. Start from the top: 10, 9, 8, 7, 6, 5....until you reach the bottom. With each step breathe in, and as you let go, breathe out, relax and feel your body become heavy and at ease. As you go down the steps you will become more relaxed, and finally drift into a meditative state. By the time you reach the bottom step you will feel completely relaxed.

As you breathe, breathe in the sun; breathe out the light, making sure the rhythm of your breath is slow and gentle. Breathe In light, and then breathe out love. Breathe in love, and then breathe out light.

Picture yourself in a special place and visualise your body in perfect health. Every cell in your body is in perfect order. You may want to visualise God and your Angels surrounding you or walking with you along the beach on a tropical island. You are surrounded with white light, and feel the sun penetrating your skin absorbing the healing benefits of vitamin D in every cell.

Spend at least ten minutes preferably 30 minutes to an hour on this activity every day. You can change your special place according to how you feel.

Centering your mind

If you have difficulty in centering your mind, light a candle. Focus on the candle and your breath for a few minutes, until you feel you would like to close your eyes. Then slowly close your eyes, keeping the image of the candle in your mind's eye. Develop your skills by adding a flower or some other object to the candle. In time your ability to visualize will improve. You will then be able to use your imagination to take you to your perfect place.

Candles

The burning candle is essential for you to concentrate and visualise. It creates a relaxed atmosphere. Candles are also lit for protection, regaining health, developing psychic powers, and for spiritual cleansings. They are found on altars and other ritual places linking to a God source.

We are fortunate to have many types of candles produced today. Make sure your candles are non-toxic. Candles made from soy, do not smoulder or give off poisons when they are blown out and they last longer.

Incense

Incense symbolizes air. As the smoke rises our thoughts are carried up into the universe.

You will need incense that is chemical-free. You will also need an incense burner. To save money, find a container or flower pot you like, and fill it with sand. Stand the incense in this container together with the candles if you like.

Frankincense, sandalwood, patchouli, and cedarwood are the best incense to light while meditating. White sage will clear the air of negative energy.

Pure Essential oils

Essential oils boost immunity as long as they are pure. Avoid cheap brands described 'fragrant oil'. Fragrant oils contain harmful chemicals. Put a couple of drops of purified essential oil in purified filtered water in an oil burner. There is no need to light incense when using essential oils.

Essential Oils can also be added to a bath to encourage relaxation. Put a few drops in a humidifier, if you own one, or on your pillow.

To create a peaceful stress free environment use clary sage, lavender, basil, chamomile, geranium, lemon, mandarin, orange, neroli, myrrh, patchouli, ylang ylang, rose thyme and bergamot.

You can use a combination of oils, or just one. Patchouli, cedarwood, sandalwood and frankincense are good oils for meditation or you could combine the following to create balance whilst meditating.

Use 5 drops frankincense, 5 drops orange or mandarin, 10 drops cedarwood, and 2 drops of rosewood. Place the mixture in a cup of water, and add it to an oil burner or diffuser.

Setting the scene

It is a good idea to dedicate a place in your home for meditation and prayer. It is also best to meditate in the same place each day and set up an Alter.

The Alter should have a flat surface. A coffee table or a timber box are suitable or even a branch off a tree if you are meditating outside. Be creative. You may like to cover the Alter with a piece of fabric, and then put your candles, incense and crystals on top.

Once you have set up your favourite place for meditation or prayer; you may find this a good place to write your affirmations as well.

Take time out daily to meditate and seek guidance.

Walks in the forest or on the beach — pure air

If you live in a city, you should try to get yourself to a beach, the country or the mountains on a regular basis. Pure fresh air is essential for your health.

Find a place where the air is clean. Oxygen is important for cellular regeneration. It is best to walk in places where the air is clean and fresh. There is less pollution by the sea or in the forest.

- Avoid smog, cigarette smoke and fumes.
- Practice deep breathing from the diaphragm.
- Take exercise in the mountains or by the sea, if possible.
- Air your bedding regularly.
- Sleep with a window or door opened for better ventilation.
- Holiday near the ocean, lakes, or in the mountains.

In less polluted areas you will be able to think more clearly, your energy levels will improve, and you will feel calmer and less stressed.

Vitamin D — Exposure to the sun

The sun is most important to healing — especially from sunrise until 10am and again after 3pm. Avoid excess exposure to the sun between these hours, especially if you live in the tropics or subtropics.

Australians and many nationalities living in the tropics and subtropics have been so brainwashed about the dangers of sun cancer that they tend to cover up all the time, and use poisonous sun screens. The dangers have been overstated in my opinion. We need the sun to synthesis vitamin D. The sun converts cholesterol found under the skin to vitamin D. Vitamin D is known to fight many cancers. For cancers like melanoma, the sun is not always an enemy. Your weakened immune system is your enemy, and your lifestyle has probably triggered your health problems.

Low vitamin D has been linked to multiple sclerosis, jaundice, cancer, PMS, arthritis, underactive thyroid, acute depression, dermatitis and many other diseases and conditions.

The sun increases the melatonin levels and synthesises them during the night. This helps to regulate sleep. Early morning walks before 10am or late afternoon walks after 3pm in the sun, without sun glasses, will help you get a good night's sleep.

Sun bathing without your clothes on, if possible, is extremely healing, and will also kill bacteria.

So get out there. Expose! Expose! Expose! (No trench coats please). Find a private spot if you can, and start with ten minutes a day. Then increase that to about twenty minutes a day. If you do not have a place to go naked, then, wear the least amount of clothing that you can, weather and climate permitting of course.

Try to avoid exposing yourself to the sun between the hours of 10am and 3pm. There is an exception to this as the latest studies say that 10-15 minutes only in the middle of the day is beneficial for the absorption of Vitamin D, especially in countries like England where the sun is not as plentiful. Use organic 30 plus sunscreen if being out in the sun at these times is unavoidable. It is important to buy only organic or chemical free sunscreens.

Temperance

By the time you have beaten cancer your taste buds will have changed dramatically, together with your way of thinking. There will be times however when you will want to step outside the box and be a little naughty. I think this is more psychological than physiological. If you do decide to dabble in a little naughty and nice, do so in moderation, and keep control of your new way of life. I do not live a life of a saint. I do however keep my indulgences down to a bare minimum. My favourite indulgence is going for a walk along the beach followed by a genuine dairy free, sugar free fruit Gelati Ice Cream. If you like ice-cream find a vendor that sells genuine fruit Gelati, very creamy very tasty. My husband Wayne and I do this once a week in summer and I look forward to it.

If going to a party or a get-together with family or friends, make one of the sweet treats in this book or find one in 'The Cancer to Wellness Cookbook'. You might be surprised at how well these treats go down with others.

I also have a glass of wine occasionally. My husband Wayne does not drink any alcohol at all; this is a blessing I guess in our home. In the past, I have enjoyed many a glass of wine. Now-a-days I can only handle one glass on very few occasions. My body has adjusted to a new way of life and I do not want to drink very often. Every now and then I will partake and enjoy one glass of red wine followed by heaps of water.

Many of us before starting a more nutritious way of life had become addicted to certain foods and beverages. Believe me when I say, your new way of nurturing your body and mind is even more addictive. Healthy living and feeling great is very addictive.

Other alternative therapies

There are many alternative healing techniques such as Reiki which can teach the art of self healing. Reiki has different levels. Reiki one, is about self healing. After you have qualified in level one you may like to study further and in more detail to be in a position to heal others.

The following therapies listed may be helpful for you: Kinesiology, Pilates, Theta Healing, Myotherapy Bowen therapy, Aromatherapy, Yoga, Breathing Therapies, Tai Chi, Aura and Chakra healing, healing with sound and colour, Crystal therapy, Laughter therapy and, Biofeedback, Bach flower remedies, Polarity Therapy, NLP, EMF Balancing Techniques. There are excellent practitioners in all these areas today.

The do's and don'ts of massage

I had enjoyed massage regularly for many years but I had to be more careful when I had cancer. Lymphatic massage is dangerous for most cancer sufferers, as it may spread the bad cancer cells through the body. I restricted myself to facial and foot massages, and I found them just as relaxing. I gave the therapist clear instructions, and made sure she or he did not go anywhere near my lymphatic system. Many practitioners now use only organic and chemical-free products. Enquire prior to booking a massage or facial to find out what products they use.

Exercise

Our immune system benefits greatly from daily exercise. It improves circulation, and helps to carry nutrients to all our organs, and eliminates waste. Exercise also stimulates the production of human growth hormone (HGH), and helps to repair muscle tissue, bones, hair, and nails, and is good for the skin and is anti aging. Exercise releases endorphins to the brain. These are the chemicals which make you feel good, and combat stress and anxiety. Exercise promotes a good night's sleep and is especially recommended for those suffering from depression.

Regular exercise improves bone density and reduces the risk of some cancers, such as breast cancer. It also lowers cholesterol and blood pressure for those who are susceptible. However, what many people do not realise is that exercise without weight-bearing exercise is counterproductive as it is important for improving bone density and strength.

If motivation is a problem, you may need a personal trainer for a while. He or she will be able to show you ways to exercise that are safe, and conducive to good health.

Personal training

Personal training has become common, no longer reserved for the rich and famous. Finding a good personal trainer qualified in rehabilitation, alignment procedures, and core stability is most important.

How to choose the right trainer

Make sure your trainer really cares about his clients, has plenty of experience, and has a background in rehabilitation. A competent trainer works to activate your core, where all movement is centred. That includes the pelvic floor. Basic body alignment principles should be the emphasis of their routines. Aerobic and cardio conditioning need to be implemented slowly if the client is extremely unfit.

Abdominal workouts are usually recommended to enhance core muscle. But there is a great deal more core work needed than that. A feeble core leaves you vulnerable to injury, lower back pain, poor balance and posture. It also leads to the wasting away of those muscles that support the pelvic floor, which produces prolapsed anal and pubic areas. Core strengthening exercises are vital for good body condition. The core is your centre of gravity.

Choose a personal trainer who will work with your physiotherapist, osteopath or chiropractor. Most people have injuries that occurred earlier in their life, and your trainer needs to know about them. Effective training will not only help those with injury, it will help to minimise or avoid any future injuries.

A weakened core probably accounts for physiotherapists and chiropractors being so busy these days and for the very high frequency of injuries in sport at all levels, even among the elite. Only the best informed coaches and trainers undertake core training for their clients. I see very few trainers using this type of training. I also suspect that many are so full of their own importance that they neglect the needs of their clients. Avoid trainers who treat you like you are an item on an assembly line. Likewise, avoid trainers who treat you as if you have just joined the army.

It is no harder to find a genuine personal trainer than a bad one. Do not settle for second best. Do not choose them just because you think he or she is cute. Watch them closely beforehand and observe if they demonstrate the qualities you are looking for in a gentle manner. Your trainer needs to be passionate, and have good people skills, and a positive attitude toward you. If you find someone with these credentials then give them a go.

Trainers who do not keep a close eye on their clients, and seem to be chewing gum and thinking about something else when they are supposed to be training should be given a wide berth. Do not go with trainers who tell you core training and basic alignment is unnecessary. There is no shortage of trainers to choose from. Just practice discernment in making your choice. Also make sure your trainer practices what they preach!

Benefits of core training (Ref: Empowering the trainer within by Wayne Matheson)

1. Provides protection for your back by strengthening the core muscles.

2. Provides core stability because of your trunk becoming stronger.

3. Stabilizes your centre of gravity.

4. Improves your posture.

5. Improves your balance.

6. Improves your shape.

7. Improves your performance during exercises and sports activities.

8. Improves your technique in strength training and therefore your strength.

9. Improves your stamina in aerobic activity.

10. Makes you less susceptible to back pain and other injuries.

11. Gives you something to focus on during long aerobic activities like running.

12. Body movements become easier.

13. Muscles work more harmoniously together.

14. Daily exercises and work will be performed with ease.

15. The core will become your source of power.

16. Better bladder control.

17. Better haemorrhoid control.

18. Greater control of the pelvic muscles which reduce prolapsing of the uterus and the vagina.

19. Helps contract hernia of the bladder, and the bowels and reduces haemorrhoids.

20. Helps control prostate enlargement.

22. Increases sexual function.

23. Improves neuro pathways.

*E*very cell, nerve,
tissue, organ and bone is
now made whole, pure
and perfect.

*M*y whole body
is being restored
to health and
harmony.

Recipes

The recipes in this book are to be integrated into your program. They will be beneficial towards your healing and your wellbeing. They are designed to ensure a high grade of necessary nutrients and are very simple to prepare.

The use of simple foods that are from organic ingredients will ensure that you have a healthy immune system and will be great for your family and friends to enjoy.

Changing your daily dietary intake may seem foreign at first, but change need not be your enemy. Change can be truly a time to free yourself of old habits that have not worked for you.

The recipes in this book are not only well balanced and good for you, they are delicious and easy to prepare.

POTASSIUM BROTH (1)

The following broth recipe will make approximately 4 litres of broth.

Ingredients:

5 large potatoes — red, white or sweet/yam, 4 large carrots, 2 large brown onions, with skin, ½ bunch celery, 1 bunch parsley, 1 nob of garlic. Add a wedge or two of pumpkin to sweeten, 1 tsp Celtic salt, Nob of fresh turmeric, 1 bunch coriander. Pure clean filtered water.

You will need one 6 litre or 6 quart (approximately) stainless steel pot with lid or crock pot.

Method:

1. Wash vegetables thoroughly and brush off any excess dirt leaving the skins on.
2. Cut ingredients and place into the large pot and cover with water.
3. Bring to boil, and then boil for ½ hour keeping the water level above the ingredients.
4. Simmer on a gentle flame or low heat for another 2 hours.
5. Let stand for no less than 30 minutes.
6. Mash ingredients gently in order for the flavours to blend.
7. Let cool and strain off pulp from broth using cheese cloth.
8. Place in glass containers or bottles and refrigerate.
9. Freeze any excess broth until ready to use. Broth will last only two days in the fridge before turning rancid.
10. Compost or discard vegetables.

Serve in a large cup. Top with a small sprinkle of Cayenne pepper (optional). **Cayenne pepper** is anti-bacterial, anti-cancer, a powerful antioxidant and a powerful circulatory stimulant. Avoid in cases of gastritis or ulcer.

The following broth recipe will make approximately 4 litres of broth.

Ingredients:

5 large potatoes — red, white, sweet/yam

4 large carrots

¼ cup cabbage

¼ cup spinach or choose from one of the following: kale, broccoli, Swiss chard or watercress, 1 bunch of parsley, ¼ cup mushrooms, ½ bunch celery, 1 cup red beets, 1 nob of garlic, 1 nob of fresh turmeric, 1 tsp Celtic salt, Add any other herbs you desire. Pure clean water.

You will need one 6 litre or 6 quart (approximately) stainless steel pot with lid or crock pot.

Method:

1. Wash vegetables thoroughly and brush off any excess dirt, leaving skins on.

2. Cut ingredients and place into the large pot and cover with water.

3. Bring to boil and then boil for ½ hour keeping the water level covering the ingredients.

4. Simmer on a gentle flame or low heat for another 2 hours.

5. Let stand for no less than 30 minutes.

6. Mash ingredients gently in order for the flavours to blend.

7. Let cool and strain off pulp from broth using cheese cloth.

8. Place in glass containers or bottles and refrigerate.

9. Freeze any excess broth until ready to use — broth will last only two days in the fridge before turning rancid.

10. Compost or discard vegetables.

Serve in a large cup. Top with a small sprinkle of Cayenne pepper (optional).

Cayenne pepper is anti-bacterial, anti-cancer, a powerful antioxidant and a powerful circulatory stimulant. Avoid in cases of gastritis or ulcer.

Juices

Process all fruit and vegetables slowly in small amounts through
a juicer nozzle, and then serve in your sexy long glass.

Add ⅓ water to ⅔ juice.

If organic fruit and vegetable are not available; place produce in water with
4 teaspoons of vinegar to eliminate excess chemicals and fertilizer residue.

WATERMELON JUICE, MINT

Ingredients:

½ watermelon

3 to 4 leaves of mint

Method:

1. Wash outside skin thoroughly.

2. Chop produce into small chunks (leaving the skin on — optional).

3. Wash leaves of mint thoroughly.

PINEAPPLE, PEAR, GINGER

Ingredients:

¼ large pineapple

2 pears

1 slice of ginger (according to taste)

Method:

1. Skin Pineapple.

2. Wash or Core Pear.

3. Wash Ginger.

KIWIFRUIT, APPLE, CELERY

Ingredients:

4 green apples

2 kiwifruit

1 celery stalk

Method:

1. Skin and core apples.

2. Wash kiwi fruit and cut into four.

3. Wash celery.

CARROT, APPLE, BEETROOT, CELERY, GINGER

Ingredients:

1 large carrot

1 large apple

1 medium beetroot

1–2 celery stalks including leaves

1 piece of ginger (size according to taste)

Method:

1. Wash and brush carrot until clean.

2. Skin and core apple.

3. Trim and brush clean beetroot.

4. Wash celery thoroughly.

5. Wash ginger.

CARROT, SPINACH, PARSLEY, PINEAPPLE

Ingredients:

½ pineapple

1 small bunch parsley

2 spinach stems

1 large carrot

Method:

1. Remove skin of pineapple.

2. Wash and brush carrot until clean.

3. Wash parsley and spinach.

CARROT, SPINACH, APPLE, TURNIP LEAVES

Ingredients:

2 large carrots

2 spinach stems

2 apples

Small bunch of turnip leaves

Method:

1. Wash and brush carrot until clean.

2. Wash spinach.

3. Skin and core apple.

4. Wash turnip leaves.

CELERY, CUCUMBER, CARROT, SPINACH

Ingredients:

2 stalks celery

1 small cucumber

2 large carrots

2 stems spinach

Method:

1. Wash and clean celery.

2. Wash and clean cucumber.

3. Wash and brush carrots until clean.

4. Wash and clean spinach.

POTATO, ENDIVE, APPLE, GINGER

Ingredients:

2 medium potatoes

Small bunch endive

2 large green apples

1 piece of ginger (according to taste)

Method:

1. Wash and brush potatoes until clean.

2. Wash endive.

3. Skin and core apples.

4. Wash ginger.

5. Cut produce into small pieces.

KALE, APPLE, BEETROOT WITH GREENS, GARLIC, CABBAGE

Ingredients:

Handful of kale

2 apples

1 medium beetroot and leaves

1 clove garlic

¼ head cabbage

Method:

1. Wash kale.

2. Wash and core apples.

3. Trim, wash and brush beetroot until clean.

4. Trim garlic.

5. Wash cabbage.

6. Cut produce into small pieces.

SPINACH, BROCCOLI, RED PEPPER, GARLIC, APPLE

Ingredients:

2 large spinach leaves

2 broccoli flowerets

1 medium capsicum

1 clove garlic

2 green apples

Method:

1. Wash spinach leaves.

2. Wash broccoli.

3. Wash capsicum.

4. Trim garlic.

5. Wash and core apples.

BEETROOT, CARROT, SPINACH

Ingredients:

1 medium beetroot

1 large carrot

2 large spinach leaves

Method:

1. Trim, wash and brush beetroot clean.

2. Wash and brush carrot clean.

3. Wash spinach leaves.

WHEAT GRASS

Wheat grass contains many anti-cancer properties such as chlorophyll, the best source of living chlorophyll available. It contains selenium, B12, B vitamins, minerals and trace elements, amino acids and over eighty active enzymes to help regenerate the body and build the immune system.

The chlorophyll in wheat grass has almost the same molecular structure as haemoglobin and increases the production of haemoglobin therefore increasing more oxygen in the body and supports the pH in the system. This helps to fight and prevent cancer.

Wheat grass has superior detoxification benefits, it purifies the liver and washes out and neutralises toxins, chemicals and drugs in the body.

Wheat grass needs to be taken in small dosages. Start with 1–2mls (1–2oz) then gradually increase to 10mls (10oz) daily. Dilute half and half with filtered water. Large doses of wheat grass can cause a healing crisis as it will dump toxins faster by speeding up detoxification.

Wheat grass juice is to be taken alone, thirty minutes prior to any other food, beverage, exercise and, enemas or colonics.

Wheat grass juice implants in enemas are also recommended during the detoxification juice program.

Ann Wigmore's book 'Be Your Own Doctor' is full of information and practical tools for sprouting wheat grass and other sprouting tips including many recipes.

BENEFITS OF JUICING

Fruit and vegetable juices build, restore and cleanse the body. They offer anti-cancer fighting anti-oxidants.

Apart from the recipes included in this handbook; you can combine sprouts, dandelion greens, chard, and watercress, broccoli with apples, carrots, onions or radishes with any of the recipes. Be creative and design your own juice recipes using the food combining chart for better digestion.

PROTEIN AND CALCIUM ENRICHED RAW FRUIT, MUESLI AND SLAPSB

Serves 1

$\mathcal{I}$ngredients:

1 cup papaya

1 kiwi fruit

6–8 large strawberries

½ punnet blueberries

You can use whatever fruit is in season as long as there is a minimum of 3 varieties and range of colour.

2 tbls SLAPSB (sunflower kernels, linseed, almonds, pumpkin seeds, sesame seeds and Brazil nuts) *see recipe next page.*

2 tbls rolled oats

1 tsp Bee pollen

1 dsp Living Valley Springs Breakfast Herbs. Begin with ¼ tsp. Gradually increase by ¼ tsp daily. These herbs are very strong in flavour and you will need time to adjust your taste buds.

¼ tsp organic maca-avoid if you have a thyroid problem.

½ cup non dairy milk: coconut, rice, almond, or oat milk.

or

Organic cahew cream, yoghurt or biodynamic yoghurt for topping.

$\mathcal{M}$ethod:

1. Wash, peel and seed papaya.

2. Wash and trim strawberries.

3. Wash and peel kiwifruit.

4. Wash blueberries.

5. Place fruit in a bowl with dry ingredients and milk.

SLAPSB

Serves 1

Ingredients:

1 tbls sunflower seeds

1 tbls linseed

½ tbls almonds

1 tbls pepitas

½ tbls sesame seeds

½ tbls Brazil nuts

Method:

Grind seeds and nuts in a grinder. A coffee grinder will do.

If you do not have a grinder soak all ingredients overnight in a little filtered water or non dairy milk.

This recipe can be made in bulk. Keep in a glass jar in the refrigerator.

To make a bulk amount, replace 1tbls with 1 cup and ½ a tbls with ½ a cup.

FRUIT SALAD AND CASHEW CREAM

Serves 1

Ingredients:

½ a banana

3 large strawberries

10 blueberries

1 kiwi fruit

½ cup papaya

Small handful of grapes

1 passion fruit

¼ cup cashew cream

Method:

1. Wash, trim, skin and cut all fruit into small pieces.

2. Place in a serving bowl.

3. Top with cashew cream.

CASHEW CREAM

Serves 1–2

Ingredients:

½ cup cashews

Enough non dairy milk to cover nuts and to blend smooth

Method:

1. Soak cashews in water in a glass bowl for at least one hour. It is best to soak them overnight.

2. Rinse off water and place cashews into a blender.

3. Add milk.

4. Blend ingredients, add milk to desired consistency

Store any leftover cream in a jar in the refrigerator. This will keep for one day.

POACHED EGGS, AVOCADO, TOMATO WITH BASIL WITH BALSAMIC AND OLIVE OIL DRESSING

Ingredients:

Eggs, Avocado & Tomato

2 eggs

½ avocado

1 roma tomato or 6 cherry tomatoes

1 tbls chopped basil

Dressing

¼ cup organic extra virgin olive oil

2 tsp balsamic vinegar

1 clove crushed garlic

Method:

Eggs, Avocado & Tomato

1. Wash tomatoes and slice into small pieces set aside.

2. Wash and finely chop basil.

3. Peel and finely slice avocado and shape into half circle set aside.

4. Place into a deep frypan, filtered water and bring almost to boil.

5. Add a little fine Celtic salt.

6. Gently crack eggs and place eggs in water, cook until desired consistency making sure they do not hard boil.

When eggs are cooked, serve on buckwheat waffles, corn bread, or sour dough bread of your choice toasted. Place eggs, avocado, tomatoes on the plate, garnish avocado and tomato with basil and a little drizzle of the prepared dressing. Add a little cayenne pepper and fine Celtic salt on the eggs according to taste.

Dressing

Put ingredients in a small jar, shake well and store in the fridge. *(This dressing will last for some time and can be used on salads.)*

POACHED EGGS WITH LVS CORIANDER CHELATION PESTO

$\mathcal{I}$ngredients:

2 poached eggs

1 slice sour dough toast

1 tbls coriander Chelation pesto

Coriander Chelation Pesto

This is a magic recipe I was given at Living Valley Springs.

4 cloves of garlic

⅓ cup Brazil nuts

⅓ cup sunflower seeds

⅓ cup pumpkin seeds

2 cups packed fresh coriander

⅔ cup extra virgin olive oil

4 tbls lemon juice

½ tsp fine Celtic salt

$\mathcal{M}$ethod:

1. Process the coriander and olive oil in the blender.

2. Add garlic, nuts, seeds, salt and lemon juice.

3. Mix until the mixture is finely blended into a paste and ready to serve.

4. Store in dark glass jar if possible in refrigerator.

5. This mixture freezes well.

Two teaspoons of this pesto a day for three to four weeks is known to remove heavy metals. Heavy metals include mercury, lead and aluminium. Coriander is an excellent blood purifier. This pesto goes well with eggs, toast, dry baked potatoes, pasta and rice.

BAKED TOMATO AND MUSHROOM STACK

Serves 2

Ingredients:

2 large egg tomatoes cut in half

4 large mushrooms washed and trimmed

1 medium red onion finely sliced

1 fennel bulb washed trimmed, and cut lengthwise into 1½ cm slices

2 large garlic cloves trimmed and cut into half

¼ cup ricotta cheese crumbled or ¼ cup crumbled soya cheese

2 tbls cold pressed olive oil

2 tsp balsamic vinegar

Handful of fresh coriander or parsley

Method:

1. Preheat oven to 200°C 15 minutes prior to using — adjust oven to 180°C when in use.

2. Arrange vegetables and cheese including garlic into two stacks on a baking sheet in a baking tray that has been slightly oil brushed.

3. Mix olive oil and balsamic, drizzle over each stack.

4. Bake in oven for 10–12 minutes or until lightly coloured.

5. Place 1 slice of your favourite sour dough toast in the centre of dinner plate.

6. Add vegetable stack.

7. Garnish with coriander or parsley.

8. Serve.

Add a couple of poached eggs and other vegetables to this dish if you desire.

SCRAMBLED TOFU

Serves 2

Ingredients:

2 cups firm tofu crumbled to the size and form of scrambled eggs

(You can do this with either your fingers or a fork.)

1 tsp coconut oil

2 tsp tamari sauce

½ tsp turmeric

½ tsp onion powder

1 red onion finely chopped

1 crushed garlic clove

1 tsp fine Celtic salt

1 tbls nutritional yeast

Handful of parsley

Method:

1. Press tofu to remove excess water. Do this by taking it out of the wrapper, place on a plate and put another plate on top and press down releasing the excess water.

2. Crumble tofu and place in a large bowl.

3. Add onion powder, turmeric, Celtic salt, nutritional yeast and tamari, set aside.

4. Place oil in a skillet or frying pan and heat over a medium heat — do not overheat.

5. Add onion and garlic — cook until onions look clear.

6. Add marinated tofu and stir around in the skillet making sure you do not burn or overcook.

7. Tofu should start to resemble scrambled eggs and take on a yellow hue. Keep cooking until all liquid evaporates.

8. Serve with sour dough bread of your choice — top with parsley.

9. Add slices of raw tomato and ½ an avocado together with salad vegetables of your choice.

ALMOND MEAL PANCAKES TOPPED WITH BERRIES & YOGHURT

Serves 1

Ingredients:

Pancake Mix

⅓ cup almond meal

1 tbls yoghurt

1 dsp Xylitol

1 egg

1 or 2 tbls water

1 tsp coconut oil

½ tsp baking soda

Yoghurt & Berry Mix

⅓ cup yoghurt

½ cup strawberries

½ cup blueberries

½ cup raspberries

1 dsp Xylitol

Method:

Pancake Mix

1. Place ingredients in a mixer and blend together.
2. Place a little coconut oil on a hot skillet.
3. Divide mixture into 3 parts and cook on hot skillet.
4. Serve on a dinner plate.
5. Top with yoghurt and berry mix.

Yoghurt & Berry Mix

1. Wash all berries.
2. Trim strawberries and cut into quarters.
3. Place Xylitol and ¼ of the berries in blender.
4. Blend until smooth.
5. Place mixture on top of pancakes and scatter remaining berries.
6. Decorate with a couple of mint leaves or coconut flakes.

Shakes & Smoothies

PINA COLADA BREAKFAST SHAKE

Ingredients:

1 cup fresh pineapple juice

1 cup coconut milk

2 tbls coconut oil

2 scoops vanilla de-natured protein powder

¼ cup ice

Leaves of mint for decorative purposes

Method:

1. Place ingredients in a blender for 15–20 seconds until frothy.

2. Serve in a long glass.

3. Top with mint.

4. Sip slowly.

PAPAYA AND ORANGE BREAKFAST SHAKE

Ingredients:

1 cup papaya

1 orange (juice only)

1 cup non dairy milk

¼ tsp pure vanilla essence

2 scoops of raw organic protein powder

The seeds of the papaya can also be used as they are very therapeutic — they are a little bitter to taste at first but one does get used to it.

Method:

1. Place all ingredients in a blender for 15–20 seconds until frothy.

2. Serve in a long glass.

3. Sip slowly.

The following smoothie I found on a web site www.alivefoods.com/recipes —according to the site the recipe comes from a former chef of His Holiness the Dalai Lama who now runs an organic market on Manhattan's East Side. I decided to try the recipe and thought the ingredients alone told the story. I hope you enjoy this recipe as much as I do. Access this site for some really good living food recipe books.

SPINACH SMOOTHIE

Ingredients:

2 spinach leaves

¼ large papaya

1 handful of parsley

1 handful of dandelion root

1 banana

Juice of 2–3 freshly squeezed oranges

Method:

1. Place ingredients in a blender and blend until smooth and frothy.

2. Serve in a tall glass.

3. Sip slowly.

SPROUTED WHEAT AND FIG SMOOTHIE

Ingredients:

¼ cup of sprouted wheat seeds

¼ cup filtered water

½ cup non dairy milk

3 figs that have been soaked overnight

Method:

1. Place ingredients in a blender and blend until smooth and frothy.

2. Serve in a tall glass.

3. Sip slowly.

SPROUTED SEEDS AND PINEAPPLE CHUNK SMOOTHIE

Ingredients:

½ cup sprouted alfalfa seeds

2 tbls sprouted sesame seeds

½ cup pineapple chunks

½ cup non dairy milk

Method:

1. Place ingredients in a blender and blend until smooth and frothy.

2. Serve in a tall glass.

3. Sip slowly.

BUCKWHEAT WAFFLES

Ingredients:

1 ⅓ cups buckwheat flour sifted twice

¾ cup filtered water

1 cup filtered hot water

½ cup cooked brown rice

½ tsp fine Celtic salt

Method:

1. Combine flour and ¾ cup of water.

2. Stir to make a paste — set aside for at least one hour.

3. Place ingredients including paste into a blender.

4. Blend thoroughly.

5. Additional water may be necessary.

6. Heat a waffle maker.

7. Place in required amounts and cook until ready.

Any waffles left over can be placed in the freezer and warmed in the toaster or oven when needed.

CORN BREAD

Ingredients:

2 cups corn kernels

2 cups filtered water

1 tsp fine Celtic salt

¼ cup cold pressed olive oil

1 cup polenta

Method:

1. Blend corn kernels and water.

2. Place into a mixing bowl.

3. Stir in salt and oil.

4. Add polenta and mix well.

5. Pour into bread tin and bake for 45–60 mins at 108°C or until firm.

When cool cut into serving sizes and place in freezer and warm in toaster or oven when needed.

CRACKER BREAD

Ingredients:

1 ½ cups sprouted wheat

Water

1 tsp Celtic salt

Herbs, spices to taste

Method:

1. Blend sprouted wheat with enough water to form a smooth fine mixture.

2. Add any herbs, Celtic salt and spices of choice or choose to keep plain.

3. Pour into a non stick biscuit tin.

4. Place in oven on a low heat around 50°C until crispy.

Or

If using a Ezi Dry De-Hydrator pour mixture thinly over dehydrator sheets.

1. Spread evenly.

2. Sprinkle chives, paprika, sesame etc on top.

3. Dry in a dehydrator at 38°C for approximately 48 hours or until bread lifts easily from sheets.

To make green bread: Blend zucchini, parsley, chives and/or broccoli with sprouted wheat and water.

To make red bread: Blend capsicum, tomatoes, paprika and/or cayenne pepper with sprouted wheat andwater.

To make Italian bread: Blend capsicum, onion, garlic, oregano, marjoram and/or basil with sprouted wheat and water.

$\mathcal{S}$alads

GARDEN SALAD

$\mathcal{I}$ngredients:

60–80g mixed lettuce, 1 grated medium carrot, 1 grated small beetroot, 6–8 cherry tomatoes or 2 roma tomatoes, ¼ medium red onion, 1 oven roasted red or green pepper, 4 semi-sundried tomatoes, 1 avocado, sprouts.

Small handful of the following: fresh basil, fresh mint, fresh flat leaf parsley, mung beans, pine nuts, sunflower seeds, and sundried sultanas (optional).

4 artichokes (optional and store bought) chopping each piece into two.

$\mathcal{M}$ethod:

1. Preheat oven to 200°C/400°F.
2. Cut peppers into half. Remove seeds and stalk and place on a baking sheet.
3. Drizzle the olive oil over peppers.
4. Crush and scatter garlic over peppers.
5. Season with Celtic salt.
6. Bake in oven for 20–25 minutes.
7. Remove and cool when cooked, cut into strips, place ½ in salad mix and ½ into refrigerator for another time.
8. Whilst peppers are cooking wash other vegetables and herbs.
9. Break lettuce into small pieces by hand. *(Do not cut with a knife)*.
10. Chop cherry tomatoes into halves.
11. Peel and grate carrot and beetroot.
12. Chop sundried tomatoes in strips.
13. Peel onions and finely slice.
14. Finely chop herbs.
15. Peel avocado, remove seed and cut into cubes.
16. Place ingredients into a large salad bowl and toss.
17. Add your choice of dressing and serve — see dressing section.

PAPAYA AND AVOCADO SALAD
WITH LIME & GINGER DRESSING

Ingredients:

Salad

4 cups chopped endive or mixed lettuce

2 cups papaya

1 large avocado

2–4 green shallots

Lime & Ginger Dressing

¼ cup olive oil

¼ cup lime juice

1 tbls grated fresh ginger

¼ tsp mild curry powder

Method:

Salad

1. Wash and chop endive.

2. Peel, seed and cut papaya into cubes.

3. Cut avocado into half remove seed and skin.

4. Chop avocado into cubes.

5. Wash, trim and finely chop shallots.

6. Place ingredients in a bowl.

7. Gently toss ingredients and add dressing.

Lime & Ginger Dressing

Combine ingredients in small container with lid and shake well.

CARROT AND BEET SALAD WITH LEMON & GINGER DRESSING

Ingredients:

Salad

4 grated carrots

1 large beetroot

Lemon & Ginger Dressing

1 piece of fresh ginger about ½" x 2" — peeled and grated

3 cloves of crushed garlic

5 tbls fresh lemon juice

2 tbls Xylitol

½ mild fresh chilli — finely chopped

Method:

Salad

1. Wash, trim and peel skin off beetroot.

2. Place in a steamer and steam for ten minutes, cool and cube beetroot.

3. Place carrot and beets into a bowl.

4. Pour dressing over carrot and beets.

5. Toss thoroughly and leave in the marinade for a couple of hours in the fridge in order for the flavours to mingle.

Lemon & Ginger Dressing

Place ingredients in a small container with lid and shake well.

MUNG BEAN AND TAMARI MUNCH

Ingredients:

2 cups mung bean sprouts

1 cup sliced brown onions

2 cloves garlic

1 tsp ginger

¼ cup tamari

⅛ cup brown rice vinegar

1 tsp sesame oil

Method:

1. Place sprouts in a colander and pour boiling water over them.

2. Sauté onions, garlic and ginger in a little water or coconut oil until onions are clear.

3. Add tamari, rice vinegar and sesame oil.

4. Simmer for 2 minutes.

5. Turn off heat, mix in the sprouts and leave for another minute.

This salad can be served also on a bed of rice together with sautéed tofu.

Dressings

AVOCADO AND TOFU DRESSING

Ingredients:

1 large avocado

½ cup silkened tofu

2 tbls cold pressed olive oil

2 tbls lemon juice

Pinch Celtic salt

¼ tsp cayenne pepper

Method:

Place ingredients in a blender and process until smooth.

Add a little water if the consistency is too thick.

BASIC VINEGARETTE

Ingredients:

¼ cup cold pressed olive oil

¼ cup white wine vinegar

1 tbls Dijon or grained mustard

1 clove of crushed garlic

1 tbls of fresh finely chopped herbs: parsley, oregano, rosemary

Method:

Place ingredients in a container with lid and shake well.

CASHEW DRESSING

Ingredients:

½ cup cashew nuts

2 tbls lemon juice

½ tsp garlic powder

½ cup water

1 pinch Celtic salt

Method:

1. Soak cashews in filtered water for at least one hour.

2. Drain off water and place in blender.

3. Add the remaining ingredients and blend until smooth.

LIME AND GINGER DRESSING

Ingredients:

¼ cup olive oil

¼ cup lime juice

1 tbls grated fresh ginger

¼ tsp mild curry powder

Method:

Combine ingredients in small container with lid and shake well until blended.

PAPAYA AND ORANGE DRESSING

Ingredients:

1 cup papaya

½ cup fresh orange juice

¼ cup lime juice

Method

Place ingredients in blender and process until smooth.

OLIVE OIL AND BALSAMIC DRESSING

Ingredients:

¼ cup cold pressed olive oil

2 tsp balsamic vinegar

1 clove crushed garlic

Method:

Place ingredients into a small container with lid and shake well.

Dips

WAYNE'S GUACAMOLE DIP

Ingredients:

2 large avocados

¼ cup lemon juice

½ small brown onion finely diced

1 large roma tomato finely chopped

1–2 tsp ground cumin

1–2 tsp ground coriander

1 clove crushed garlic

Method:

Place ingredients in a bowl and mash together.

This dip can be served with crackers, used as a salad topping and on top of dry baked vegetables.

SPROUTED HUMMUS DIP

Ingredients:

1 ½ cups of dry chickpeas (garbanzo beans)

¼ cup tahini

¼ cup cold pressed olive oil

1 cup lemon juice

3 cloves crushed garlic

1 tsp Celtic salt

1 tsp paprika

2 tbls finely chopped parsley for decoration and taste

Extra olive oil for serving

Method:

1. Soak peas for 24 hours and place in a glass jar with gauze or mesh on top. *(See Sprouting section).*

2. Wash peas and place jar upside down to drain off water.

3. Rinse daily until peas have sprouted and sprouts are about 1 ½ cm (½") in length. This usually takes 2 to 3 days.

4. When sprouts are ready place in a glass heat resistant bowl.

5. Boil kettle and let stand for 1 to 2 minutes.

6. Pour water over the peas and let stand for 1 minute. *(This is an important procedure and if not adhered to will make the hummus taste terrible.)*

7. Place peas and the other ingredients in a blender and process until smooth adding a little water if necessary.

Serve in a large bowl making a hole in the centre. Place some olive oil in the middle. Sprinkle hummus with parsley and paprika.

This dip goes well as a dressing or served with julienne vegetables, Turkish bread, wholemeal or rye pita toasted, or rice biscuits and crackers.

Sauces

HOMEMADE TOMATO SAUCE

Ingredients:

10 ripe tomatoes

2 tbls olive oil

4 garlic cloves

¼ cup tomato paste

½ tsp Celtic salt

1 tsp Xylitol

Method:

1. Puree ingredients in a food processor until smooth.

2. Store in a glass container until required.

MOCK CHEESE SAUCE

Ingredients:

1 ½ cups rice or oat milk

2 tbls olive oil

2 tbls white spelt flour

2 tbls savory yeast flakes

Method:

1. Heat oil in pan — do not burn.

2. Add flour and mix well on a low heat.

3. Add milk and stir continually. If mixture is too thick add more milk.

4. Turn off heat and add savory yeast flakes.

YOGHURT MINT SAUCE

Ingredients:

200g plain sheep yoghurt

2 tbls freshly chopped mint

2 tbls lemon juice

½ tsp Celtic salt

Method:

1. Place ingredients in a blender and process until smooth.

2. Refrigerate until required.

This sauce is great over vegie burgers, vegie slices and patties.

SAVORY CASHEW CREAM SAUCE

Ingredients:

½ cup cashews presoaked minimum 1 hour

2 cups pure water

1 tbls olive oil

2 tbls onion flakes

1 tsp celery salt

2 tbls corn flour

1 tsp vegie stock

Method:

1. Mix all ingredients in a food processor.

2. Place ingredients in a saucepan on a medium heat, stirring until smooth.

Add more liquid if needed according to required thickness.

This recipe goes well as a topping on vegetables such as asparagus, zucchini, and squash etc.

POTATO AND LENTIL PIE ITALIANA

$\mathcal{I}$ngredients:

Pastry

1 cup plain spelt flour

1 cup self raising spelt flour

½ cup (approximately) warm water

Pinch of Celtic salt

¼ cup olive oil or butter

Filling

2 cans lentils (or cook your own to the equivalent)

1 cup cooked brown rice

1 large onion diced

½ red capsicum finely diced

6 medium sized button mushrooms diced

1 large grated carrot

1 medium zucchini diced

½–1 cup parsley

2 cans diced tomatoes

2-3 tbls tomato paste

1–1 ½ cups water

2 tsp Celtic salt, 2–3 garlic cloves, 2 tbls vegie stock powder or 2 vegie stock cubes (chemical free or organic), 1–2 tsp oregano, 1–2 tsp rosemary, 1–2 tsp sage ¼ cup finely grated parmesan cheese (optional).

Topping

6 large white potatoes peeled

1 tsp Celtic salt

¼ cup oat milk

1 tbls olive oil or Butter

Paprika to sprinkle on top

Also needed: 1 Large Deep Pie Dish or 1 Large Deep Non Stick Springform Cake Tin.

$\mathcal{M}$ethod:

Pastry

1. Grease pie dish and sprinkle a little flour onto the dish.
2. Sift flour and Celtic salt into a bowl.
3. Rub in oil or butter until mixture becomes crumbly.
4. Gradually add enough water so ingredients will cling together.
5. Turn out on a floured board or surface; knead pastry until smooth.
6. Roll out pastry until 3mm thick.
7. Place pastry into greased dish or tin.
8. Set aside.

Filling

1. Heat a little coconut oil or water in a deep saucepan.
2. Add onion, garlic and capsicum and fry on a medium heat until onion softens.
3. Add mushroom, sauté for about 2–3 minutes stirring constantly.
4. Add tomatoes, water and tomato puree stir constantly.
5. Add carrot, zucchini, salt, vegie stock and herbs.
6. Add lentils and rice to the mixture.
7. Simmer for 30–45 minutes then turn off heat and set aside.

Topping

1. Place potatoes and salt in a saucepan with enough water to cover the potatoes.
2. Bring pan to boil then simmer until potatoes are soft.
3. Drain off water.
4. Add milk and oil or butter.
5. Mash until smooth.

Place filling into prepared pie dish, add parmesan (optional) and top with mashed potato. Mock cheese sauce can also be used instead of the parmesan cheese.

Sprinkle paprika on top and a little parmesan if desired.

Bake in an oven at 200°C (400°F) for 35–45 minutes or until topping is lightly browned. Let pie sit for 10 minutes before serving. Serve with large salad.

CHICKPEA PATTIES

Ingredients:

2 x 400g cans chickpeas

2 large potatoes cooked and mashed

1 grated medium carrot

1 medium onion finely diced

1–2 cloves garlic

⅓ cup coriander or parsley

1 tbls vegie stock powder

20g ground sunflower seeds

2 tbls tahini

1 egg (optional)

¼ cup polenta flour for dusting

Method:

1. Combine ingredients in a bowl and mash together.

2. Scoop half a cup of mixture out and mould with hands to make a round bulky patty.

3. Dust with a little polenta flour.

4. Pre-cook patties in a little oil in a frying pan.

5. Remove and place on a baking tray in the oven and bake for about 20 minutes.

Serve with a salad and top each patty with a little sheep's yoghurt.

WALNUT BURGERS

Ingredients:

1 cup finely ground walnuts

1 cup cooked brown rice or 1 cup ground quick oats

¼ cup spelt flour

1 cup fresh homemade breadcrumbs

½ tsp Celtic salt

½ tsp sage

1–2 cloves garlic

1–2 tsp vegie stock powder

3 tbls almond butter

2 tbls soy sauce

1 cup hot water — leave out if using rice in this recipe.

Method:

1. Mix ingredients together and let sit for at least 15 minutes before cooking.

2. Scoop ¼ cup of mixture to make one patty.

3. Cook each patty over medium heat until brown on both sides.

Serve with fresh tomato sauce and large garden salad.

To make breadcrumbs either soak bread in a little water, wring out dry, then crumble in your fingers or place bread in mill grinder until bread resembles crumbs.

NUT AND BEAN HERB LOAF

Ingredients:

½ cup hazelnuts finely ground

1 cup dry roasted cashews finely ground

1 ½ cups cooked sweet potatoes

1 can red kidney beans

1 large onion finely diced

2 eggs

¼ cup crumbled feta cheese

1 garlic clove

½ cup fresh homemade breadcrumbs

2 tbls white spelt flour

1 tbls tahini

1 tsp Celtic salt

1 tbls stock powder, 1 tsp freshly chopped thyme, 1 tsp freshly chopped rosemary, 1 tsp freshly chopped sage, ¼ tsp ground coriander, 2 tbls chopped chives, 1 tbls freshly chopped parsley

Extra flour for dusting

1 bread tin lightly greased

Method:

1. Mix ingredients together and let sit for 15 minutes before cooking.

2. Pre-heat oven to 190°C (375°F).

3. Line bread tin with baking paper.

4. Spread mixture in pan and bake in oven for 1 hour or until firm.

Serve with yoghurt mint sauce and large salad.

LENTIL AND SPINACH CASSEROLE

Ingredients:

2 cups cooked brown lentils

5 large leaves spinach roughly chopped

1 tbls olive oil

1–2 large onions

1 capsicum

1 medium carrot diced

2 large potatoes cubed

1–2 cups peeled and chopped tomatoes

1 tbls tomato paste

1 tbls fresh lemon juice

2 garlic cloves, 1 heaped tsp Celtic salt, 2 tsp ground coriander, ¼ tsp asafetida powder, ¼ tsp cayenne pepper, 1 tbls vegie stock powder, 2 tbls fresh parsley, 1 tsp xylitol

Water

Method:

1. Heat olive oil in pan and add salt, coriander, asafetida powder, cayenne pepper, xylitol, sauté for about ½ minute on high heat remove and set aside.

2. In a large pan heat a little oil and sauté onions, garlic and capsicum.

3. Add tomato and tomato puree.

4. Add all vegetables except spinach.

5. Add spices and lemon juice — stir for ½ minute over medium heat.

6. Add lentils.

7. Add enough water to cover all vegetables and lentils.

8. Simmer for an hour or two keeping the water level up.

9. Turn off heat and add parsley and chopped spinach.

10. Let stand for five minutes.

Serve in soup bowl or spaghetti bowl with large side salad and cracker bread.

CHICKPEA CASSEROLE

Ingredients:

2 x 400g canned chickpeas

1 tbls olive oil

1–2 large onions

1 capsicum

2 garlic cloves

1 medium carrot diced

2 large potatoes cubed

1–2 cups peeled and chopped tomatoes

1 tbls tomato paste

1 heaped tsp Celtic salt, 1 tbls vegie stock powder, tbls fresh parsley, 1–2 tsp ground oregano, 1–2 tsp ground rosemary, 1–2 tsp ground sage

Water

Method:

1. In a large pan heat a little oil and sauté onions, garlic and capsicum.

2. Add tomato and tomato puree.

3. Add herbs–stir for ½ minute over medium heat.

4. Add vegetables.

5. Add chickpeas.

5. Add enough water to cover all vegetables and peas.

7. Simmer for an hour or two keeping the water level up.

8. Turn off heat and let stand for five minutes.

Serve in soup bowl or spaghetti bowl.

Serve with large green side salad and cracker bread.

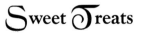

RAW CASHEW & MACADAMIA VEGAN MOCK CHEESE CAKE

Ingredients:

Pie Crust

2 cups macadamia nuts

½ cup pitted dates

¼ cup desiccated coconut

Filling

2 cups cashews–soaked overnight

¼ cup lemon juice

¼ cup agave juice

¼ cup warmed coconut oil

1 tsp pure vanilla essence

½ cup of water

Topping

1 bag of frozen raspberries or 2 punnets fresh raspberries freeze overnight.

½ cup pitted dates

Method:

Pie Crust

1. Process the macadamia nuts and dates in the food processor.

2. Sprinkle coconut onto the bottom of 8" or 9" spring form pan. This is to prevent sticking.

3. Press crust mixture onto coconut — set aside.

Filling

1. Rinse cashews and place in blender.

2. Add lemon juice, agave, vanilla, coconut oil and ½ cup of water, blend until smooth.

3. Pour mixture onto pie crust.

4. Remove any air bubbles by tapping the pan on a table.

5. Place in freezer until firm.

6. Remove whole pie and place on a serving platter.

7. Top with raspberry topping.

8. Place in refrigerator to defrost and ready to serve.

Topping

Process raspberries and dates in food processor until well blended. *(Do not use a blender for this as the raspberry seeds will become like sand.)*

Can be served with a little cashew cream or almond cream or homemade sugar free, dairy free vanilla ice cream.

This recipe was given to me by a friend. I am not sure where she got it from, but I have used it on many occasions with great success.

TRUFFLES

Ingredients:

2 cups walnuts

1 cup pitted dates

1 tbls coconut oil

3 tbls carob powder

¼ cup dessicated coconut

Method:

1. Place ingredients in a food processor.

2. Process until ingredients have blended together.

3. Scoop out small amounts to roll into small balls and roll in coconut.

4. Refrigerate until required.

FRUIT ICE CREAM

Ingredients:

Frozen lady finger bananas or frozen strawberries, mangos, kiwi fruit, melons

Method:

1. Cut pieces of fruit into small pieces and freeze.

2. Using blank screen put frozen fruit through juicer.

Bananas particularly come out thick and creamy.

SPROUTING FOR HEALTH

The way to health and longevity is to consume mostly organic raw fruits and vegetables together with a balanced amount of protein, live cultures and live produce in the form of sprouts.

Sprouts are a living food that releases and supplies energy to all the cells in the body. They are anti-aging; contain a balance of hormones both male and female that is easily assimilated in the body and are recognized for their high level of enzyme activity when they reach a stage of maturity. Processed foods lack all the vitamins and minerals our body requires to live a long healthy life.

The most essential enzymes in sprouts are amylase, protease, lipase, coagulase, emulsion, and invertase.

Vegetarians need to increase their intake of vitamin B12 and iron. Sprouts are the way to achieve this. Meats such as beef and liver that contain high levels of B12 and iron lose over 85 per cent of these vitamins when cooked.

Hardly any of the world's population eats raw meat. It is unrealistic to propose, as some do, that raw meat is the only satisfactory source of B12 and iron. Why do so many people who eat meat suffer from pernicious anemia?

Vegetarians also suffer from pernicious anemia. This is because many people have become vegetarians, not because of their awareness of nutrition issues or a desire to keep healthy; they have reacted against cruel treatment of animals. They are largely unaware of the basics of good health.

I have met many vegetarians who are obese, and suffer problems with their health. They do not have a balanced diet, and eat processed foods containing sugar and fat. They also do not exercise.

Sprouting mung beans, lentils, almonds, chickpeas and green peas will give you substantial amounts of vitamin B12. Sesame seeds, sunflower seeds, dulse or kelp and spinach increase iron.

The following seeds, grains and legumes can be sprouted:

SEEDS

Alfalfa, broccoli, celery, clover, oats, radish, fenugreek, pepitas, sunflower seeds.

GRAINS

Buckwheat, barley, millet, rice, wheat.

LEGUMES

Chickpeas, lentils, mung beans, soy beans.

NUTS

Almonds, cashews, Hunza walnuts, pecans, pistachios.

It is so easy to grow your own vegetables, even if you live in a unit, townhouse, or an apartment.

All you need for sprouting is the right equipment. Not much is required for sprouting. Buy a readymade kit that includes seeds such as a Dome Sprouter, Tray Sprouter, Jar Sprouter and Stand. These are available from www.greenharvest. com.au. Alternatively obtain glass jars with a capacity of 2 litres and with a wide mouth. Also obtain fly screen gauze, cheesecloth, or nylon from panty hose or stockings cut to size for lids, and a few rubber bands to fix the lid to the jar.

How to Sprout

- In the jar place two to four tablespoons of seeds or grains. Do not mix them as they reach maturity at different times.

- Cover with pure filtered water, filling the jar half-way.

- Place gauze over the top, and seal with a rubber band.

- Soak for at least six hours.

- Drain, rinse and turn the jar upside down to drain. This prevents rotting.

- Rinse with pure filtered water twice a day.

- Germination will take place, and seeds and grains will expand by about eight times. Keep this in mind when adding them to the jar. Legumes and nuts will not expand at the same rate. Place one cup of legumes or nuts in a jar and fill it with water. Soak no less than 15 hours. Keep washing and draining seeds, grains, legumes and nuts twice a day even after germination begins until they are ready to eat.

NB: Only use organic seeds, legumes, grains and nuts for sprouting. Non organic produce contain chemicals and may not sprout.

Congratulations if you have taken proactive and positive steps to improving your health and wellbeing. After all it is your responsibility to translate thoughts into action. Success starts with the power of intent.

My intention has been to give you the tools to live a long and fruitful life, and an understanding of how nature and our mind can cure disease.

I wish you all well. If you stick to the program you can accomplish your goals for health, happiness and longevity.

There is nothing new in this handbook except the way it has been put together: an easy step by step program to beat cancer. Everything has been tried and tested, not just by me but others seeking the same outcome — LIFE!

Love and Light. Stay true to yourself.

May you seek and find all the answers you require and be open to receive the blessings and the light of your Creator and your Guardian Angels.

Be Happy, Healthy and Prosperous.
'Seek and ye shall find.'

Kristine S. Matheson

For 24 years I have been blessed to have access to books about health, healing and spiritual practices. The time I have spent on research and self-healing has enabled me to put together this handbook. It is important that I acknowledge some of the sources of my knowledge. The following is a small selection of books I have read on my journey toward health and longevity. Included in the following selection are magazines and associations I subscribe to, DVDs and CDs, and healing centers that have influenced my life.

Books

Your Body's Many Cries for Water

F Batmanghelidj

Back to Eden

Jethro Kloss

Survival in the 21st Century

Viktoras Kulvinskas

Fats that Heal, Fats that Kill

Udo Erasmus

Nutritional Healing

Phyllis A Balch, CNC

Silent Killers

P M Taubert

Cancer-Causing Chemicals

Consumers Association of Penang

Read the Label, Know the Risk

P M Taubert

The Chemical Maze Shopping Companion — Your Guide to Food Additives and Cosmetic Ingredients

Bill Statham

Healing with Herbs and Home Remedies

Hanna Kroeger

Aromatherapy Workbook

Shirley Price

The Science and Practice of Iridology

Bernard Jensen, DCND

The Healing Mind

Dr Irving Oyle

The Sprouting Book

Ann Wigmore

Be Your Own Doctor

Ann Wigmore

Cancer — Step outside the Box

Ty Bollinger

The Nutrient Bible

Henry Osiecki

Healing With Whole Foods

Paul Pitchford

The Yeast Connection

William G Crook, MD

Virgin Coconut Oil

Brian & Marianita Jader Shilhavy

Root Canal Cover Up

George E Meinig, DDS, FACD

The pH Miracle

Dr Robert Young, PDD & Shirley Redford Young

It's All In Your Head

Dr Hal A Huggins

The Cancer Therapy

Max Gerson

Healing the Gerson Way

Charlotte Gerson with Beate Bishop

Take Control of Your Health

Elaine Hollingsworth

Dead Doctors Don't Lie

Dr Joel Wallach

Laugh With Health

Manfred Urs Kock

The Holy Bible

Includes the Eight Laws of Health

Love is Letting Go Of Fear

Gerald G Jampolsky, MD

You Can Heal Your Life

Louise L Hay

Meditations to Heal Your Life

Louise L Hay

The Power of Your Subconscious Mind

Joseph Murphy, PhD, DD

Our Emotional Links To Disease

Gregory Neville, ND

Hands of Light

Barbara Ann Brennan

Life was never meant to be a struggle

Stuart Wilde

Healing with the Angels

Doreen Virtue

The Long Road Turns to Joy — A Guide to Walking Meditation

Thich Nhat Hanh

The Voice of Silence

H P Blavatsky

Sacred Contracts

Carolyn Myss

Creating Health

Deepak Chopra

Ageless Body, Timeless Mind

Deepak Chopra

10 Secrets for Success and Inner Peace

Dr Wayne W Dyer

A Course in Miracles

Foundation for Inner Peace

Women in Silence

Grace Adamson-Gawler

Embracing the Warrior

Dr Karen Coates & Vincent Perry

I Am Grateful

Terces Engelhart with Orchid

Books

Findhorn Foundation Events and Workshops Calendar

www.findhorn.org

Hay House Events

www.hayhouse.com/events

Dr Mercola Newsletter

www.mercola.com

Cafe Gratitude Events & Workshops

www.cafegratitude.com

White Light Magazine

www.whitelightmagazine.com

The Environmental Magazine

www.emagazine.com

Living Valley Springs Lifestyle Excellence

Subscribe: free magazine or visit website www.lvs.com.au

The Relaxation Centre

www.relaxationcentreqld.com.au

The Vegetarian/Vegan Society

Google vegetarian society in your country of origin

The United Nations

Google United Nations in your country of origin

Living Now

www.livingnow.com.au

The Lucis Trust

Incorporating-The Arcane School, Triangles, World Goodwill

Suite 54, Whitehall Court, London, SW1A 2EF, United Kingdom

120 Wall Street, 24th Floor, New York, N.Y. 10005, USA

Case Postale 31, 1 Rue De Verembe (3E), 1211 Geneva 20, Switzerland

www.lucistrust.org

Subscriptions & Associations

DVDs

Feeling Great

Gary Martin, ND

This DVD covers the latest lectures by Gary Martin filmed 2008 at Wanaka, New Zealand. 10 hours viewing. Case Studies and facts that will help you optimize vitality. Purchase direct from Living Valley Springs.

The Illuminated Chakras

Judith Anodea

A visionary voyage that takes you on a multi-sensory journey into the mystical beauty of the inner world.

Health through Nutrition (Video)

Dr Joel Robbins

Food Matters

www.foodmatters.tv

CDs

Cantiones Sacrae

Findhorn Foundation

Energy and Motivation

Glenn Harold, MBSCH Dip CH

Angel Helpers

Inner World Music

Letting Go of Anxiety

Sarah Edelman

Meditations with Angels

Martine Salerno

Chakra Meditation Music

Carolyn Myss

Back Into the Universe Meditation Music

Chunyi Lin

River of Stars

Pamela and Randy Copus

The Gerson Institute

P.O. Box 161358

San Diego, CA 92176

(888) 443-7766

www.gerson.org info@gerson.org

Findhorn Foundation

Spiritual Community and Education, Eco Village

Forres. Scotland

+44 (0) 1309 690311

www.findhorn.org

Hay House Inc

P.O. Box 5100

Carlsbad, California 92018-5100

(800) 654-5126 Ext 2 United States

(760) 431-7695 Ext 2 International

www.hayhouse.com

Living Valley Springs

Kin Kin

Queensland Australia

+61 7 548 54344

www.lvs.com.au

Hippocrates Health Institute

West Palm Beach, Flordia

1800 842 2125

www.hippocratesinst.org

info@hippocratesinst.org

Alternative Healing Centre Resources

American Holistic Health Association

A selection of organic and biodynamic certifiers are:

IFOAM — International Federation of Organic Agriculture Movements. Google for organic directory online to access all international certifications.

BFA — Biological Farmers of Australia.

NASAA — National Association for Sustainable Agriculture Australia.

OHGA — Organic Herb Growers Association.

GOCA — Guaranteed Organic Certification Agency.

USDA — United States Department of Agriculture (certification agency).

OFG — Organic Farmers and Growers.

BDA — Biodynamic Agricultural Association of Australia.

ACO — Australian Certified Organic

CCOF — California Certified Organic Farmers

ACA — Accredited Certifiers Association, Inc.

BDAA — Biodynamic Agricultural Association

OFF — Organic Food Federation

FOG/QCS — Florida Organic Growers/Quality Certification Services

BDIH - Certified Natural Cosmetics Germany.

Nutritional Supplements, Raw Foods, Cafes Plus

If you live in an area where you are unable to buy what you need or you do not have a reliable holistic health care pracitioner you can go to my site www. cancertowellness. Click on Doctors & Support. This will lead you to Jack at the Broadbeach Compound Pharmacy - you will need then click on www.ewell.com. and follow the prompts. You can also email them for more information info@ewell.com.au or phone Jack on +61 7 56770562. This pharmacy will send orders wordwide.

Nature's Way Organic Vitamin C www.iherb.com Use Code HES527 to get $5 off your first order.

Gano Excel Organic Tea, coffee, toothpaste and nutritional supplements google Gano Excel in your country of origin.

Coconut Nut Oil, & various health products google www.thaiorganiclife.com

Cafe Gratitude This chain of raw food cafes are located througout California.

 Go to www.cafegratitude.com Cafe Gratitude also run workshops, food preparation classes and hold many events. They also have a helpful online shop with a wonderful raw recipe book called 'I am Grateful'.

Raw Protein Powders

www.rawpower.com, www.gardenoflife.com, www.iherb.com

What is the world offering:

If looking for raw food and/or organic cafes thoughout the world, just google Raw Food Cafes in the country of origin you either live in or are visiting. You will be surprised just how many are out there.

I would like to send much love, light and gratitude to my husband Wayne for his compassion, understanding, and unconditional love that he has given me throughout some very stressful and unsettling times. His support through my journey of self discovery and his never ending faith in me has helped me to succeed where I may have sometimes wondered what my life purpose truly was. I am so lucky to share a special love and bond with you. Also for your tireless work in order to support me whilst I wrote and published this book.

Blessings to each
and everyone.
May you be bestowed
with good health
faith and
true happiness.
— K.M.

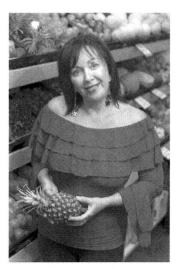

Kristine Matheson is the co- founder of The Forgotten Secrets Foundation. The foundation supports holistic education to prevent disease and to relieve sickness. She is a cancer survivor, natural nutritionist, seminar and workshop facilitator, Reiki practitioner, Angel intuitive, artist, and is a motivational and inspirational speaker.

She is the recipient of The International Women's Day 'Outstanding Inspirational Role Model Award 2011'. She has also been nominated for 'Who's Who of Australian Women 2011-2012'.

Over the years, Kristine has endured chronic fatigue, anxiety attacks, business stress, and sadly the loss of a child. These life lessons have been instrumental in her passion to treat the cause of disease.   Now, with over twenty-six years experience in natural nutrition, affirmations, and meditation, Kristine guides, and supports many people on a daily basis within her community, and throughout the world. She has made a very significant contribution to preventing and conquering cancer.

She has appeared on Today Tonight Adelaide, Nine News and many radio programs both nationally and regionally throughout Australia, and featured in regional, national, and international magazines, and newspapers, contributed to many E-newsletters, and other publications. One such publication is Olivia Newton-John's cookbook 'Livwise'.

Kristine is a very compassionate person, who has maintained a great sense of humour. She sings, dances, and is an award winning interior designer, and clothing designer. 'Singing, dancing, meditation, and exercise together with eating lots of raw live food is anti-aging' says Kristine.

Cancer changed Kristine's life for the best. Together with her husband Wayne, and several holistic medical doctors, she regularly facilitates wellness seminars. Her efforts in the community do not stop here. Kristine holds cancer support groups, plus weight loss challenges for charity incorporating Kristine's healthy food knowledge with Wayne's safe personal training and mind body techniques.

Kristine lives with her husband Wayne Matheson on the Gold Coast, Australia.

About the Author

➢ "In early 2010, I was in Australia fundraising for my wellness centre and someone gave me a book to read called 'From Cancer to Wellness: the forgotten secrets'. - I could not put it down. I was so impressed with her book and her thoughts on raw food that I immediately asked if she would contribute some of her recipes and she kindly has". **Olivia Newton-John**

➢ "Thank you for delivering your book to me personally, and all the help you provided – I was in a state of panic when we met. Your book was easy to read and even with my language difficulties, I was able to understand. It took me only five months to be very healthy again thanks to you and the information in your wonderful book. Krissy, my face is like peaches and cream all the scaring is gone." **Marie Axmann**. (Marie is French)

➢ I look forward to receiving my copy of your book "Cancer to Wellness". I don't have any serious health problems (other than minor skin cancers & hypertension). I have heard of your book from a friend of mine Peter Barnett who has followed your guidelines and gone into remission from prostate cancer. Kind regards **Richard Baxter**.

➢ "I just wanted to say thank you, I heard you on the radio last year talking about your struggle with cancer and for some strange reason I went out and purchased your book. Several months later my husband was diagnosed with Prostate Cancer after his biopsy came back positive from a T.U.R.P. operation, no need to tell you how we felt, and my husband was ready to sign the dotted line, but for some reason , maybe because we were so shocked the doctor told us to go home and think about it. We did, my husband read your book that night, decided to do it your way. Four months later, his PSA reading is 0.3 down from 3.9 no **more** mention of operation and specialist. The program helped me too (I did it with Hubby to make life easier) I lost excess weight that was refusing to budge and we both feel much healthier, thank you, thank you, thank you". **Lorna Barnett**.

- "I just finished reading your From Cancer to Wellbeing book and all I can say is...wow! I could not put it down! By upgrading every system in your body to optimum health, you could actually eliminate our most feared diseases. Seems like a daunting task, doesn't it? But that's where your book really succeeds. It is not just one of the best health books I've ever read, but also one of the easiest to digest and put into practice. Your book has changed how I will **treat** my body for the rest of my life**.** You're such an inspiring person!" **Kristine Kordic.**

- "So great chatting with you last weekend, **I found it so inspiring** that first you went the natural healing road for yourself, and then to now take it out to the world and teach what you've discovered. I read your book, and felt like there was so much value in it; it is very comprehensive and does as you say cover more than just nutrition. (Meditation, affirmations, body scrapping, sun baking etc.)". **Anthony**

- "Kris, we had a chat a few months ago. My husband Dave has the prostate cancer that had spread...Thanks to your program and his amazing 'strength' in 8 weeks his PSA has reduced from 6.3 to 3.2 – it was increasing rapidly, so now the specialist is fascinated! Just thought you would like to know. So pleased I met you and bought your book, I just felt it was going to play a big part in the story". **Carol Robinson** (this was a text message sent)

- "My name is Orannoch Campbell you can call me Nooch. I'm 28 years old, married with two children, and live in Thailand. I found out I have 6 cm brain tumour. I would like to thank you so much for your strong spirit and passing the most difficult time, and make it very good use for other people. It inspires me so much, which make me want to give you big hug and kiss if you don't mind". **Nooch**.

- "I'm not finished reading your wonderful book yet, and I just had to write to you to say, Thanks! I am really enjoying it and you have set things out very simply for readers to understand. Regards **Barry**

- "I have read your book From Cancer to Wellness, quite a journey you have been on and the information in the book is a fantastic contribution to cancer health. Sincere Regards **Bruce**.

> Hi Kristine, Loved your book, it was simple to follow without being too technical. Have CFS now for 21 yrs….been doing pretty much all that you mention in the book. It is good how you mention the brand names of Vitamins etc….. that make it so easy for sick people not to have to go around searching and buying inferior products. Thank you again and good luck with everything, and I hope you continue to enjoy all the good things in life…particularly good health." **Nia**

> I first met Kris Matheson through a "Health and Fitness" programme with a group that I attended for 3 months. I was extremely stressed, had very high blood pressure and high cholesterol. I had previously had surgery for malignant breast cancer and also suffered a prolapsed disc in my lower back (which prevented me from doing all forms of exercise). Kris was my mentor and my friend. She guided me, a unconfident sick woman with nutritional advice and knowledge. She was loving and caring and was unconditionally there for me through my struggle to get well as well as losing weight to help me with my conditions. She spent hours giving me counselling and just talking. Because of Kris's help, I now have normal blood pressure, know how to manage my back and unbelievably I am walking jogging, and exercising. WOW. I am more confident in myself and do not have stress in my life or fear a recurrence of the cancer. Kris is a bright light and a shining star an angel. Thank you Kris.. You have given my life back to me. Love Joy Clarke

Dr Carlos Orozco BSc, MSc, ND, PhD, Adv Dip Nutr, in a testimonial wrote; **"The answer to conquer and prevent cancer is in nutrition.** Very few people are aware of this. Nutrition needs to be and provided at the soul, spirit, emotional and physical level. This means we need to nourish our souls, mind, spirit and body with quality daily nutrition. **Kristine Matheson** has made a very significant contribution to preventing and conquering cancer by spreading the word through her book about the importance of nutrition in keeping a healthy body and in most cases restoring harmony into people's lives by means of daily nutrition. To do so, she shares her experience in her book entitled **From Cancer to Wellness the forgotten secrets:** A 28 day step-by-step handbook for beating cancer all based on daily nutrition for the body".

CPSIA information can be obtained at www.ICGtesting.com
Printed in the USA
LVOW051612290512

283769LV00006B/151/P